Coping with Rheumati

Dr Keith Souter is a part-time doctor, medi
Fellow of the Royal College of General Practitioners, an accredited medical acupuncturist and a specialist in homeopathic medicine. He has written a weekly health column for many years and has authored nine medical books, several of which have been translated into six languages. He takes a completely holistic and pragmatic approach to health, which is mirrored in his medical practice and in the advice on self-help which he gives in this book. In his spare time he writes novels under his own and a couple of pen-names.

Overcoming Common Problems Series

Selected titles

A full list of titles is available from Sheldon Press, 36 Causton Street, London SW1P 4ST and on our website at www.sheldonpress.co.uk

Asperger Syndrome in Adults
Dr Ruth Searle

Backache: What you need to know
Dr David Delvin

The Cancer Survivor's Handbook
Dr Terry Priestman

Coping Successfully with Prostate Cancer
Dr Tom Smith

Coping Successfully with Psoriasis
Christine Craggs-Hinton

Coping When Your Child Has Cerebral Palsy
Jill Eckersley

Coping with Birth Trauma and Postnatal Depression
Lucy Jolin

Coping with Chemotherapy
Dr Terry Priestman

Coping with Epilepsy in Children and Young People
Susan Elliot-Wright

Coping with Headaches and Migraine
Alison Frith

Coping with Life after Stroke
Dr Mareeni Raymond

Coping with Life's Challenges: Moving on from adversity
Dr Windy Dryden

Coping with Phobias and Panic
Professor Kevin Gournay

Coping with PMS
Dr Farah Ahmed and Dr Emma Cordle

Coping with the Psychological Effects of Cancer
Professor Robert Bor, Dr Carina Eriksen and Ceilidh Stapelkamp

Coping with Rheumatism and Arthritis
Dr Keith Souter

Coping with Snoring and Sleep Apnoea
Jill Eckersley

Coping with Type 2 Diabetes
Susan Elliot-Wright

Dynamic Breathing: How to manage your asthma
Dinah Bradley and Tania Clifton-Smith

The Fibromyalgia Healing Diet
Christine Craggs-Hinton

A Guide to Anger Management
Mary Hartley

How to Live with a Control Freak
Barbara Baker

How to Lower Your Blood Pressure: And keep it down
Christine Craggs-Hinton

How to Manage Chronic Fatigue
Christine Craggs-Hinton

Hysterectomy: Is it right for you?
Janet Wright

Living with Angina
Dr Tom Smith

Living with Bipolar Disorder
Dr Neel Burton

Living with Fibromyalgia
Christine Craggs-Hinton

Living with Gluten Intolerance
Jane Feinmann

Living with Physical Disability and Amputation
Dr Keren Fisher

Living with a Stoma
Professor Craig A. White

Living with Type 1 Diabetes
Dr Tom Smith

Menopause in Perspective
Philippa Pigache

Osteoporosis: Prevent and treat
Dr Tom Smith

Overcome Your Fear of Flying
Professor Robert Bor, Dr Carina Eriksen and Margaret Oakes

Overcoming Panic and Related Anxiety Disorders
Margaret Hawkins

Self-discipline: How to get it and how to keep it
Dr Windy Dryden

Sinusitis: Steps to healing
Dr Paul Carson

Understanding Traumatic Stress
Dr Nigel Hunt and Dr Sue McHale

When Someone You Love Has Dementia
Susan Elliot-Wright

Overcoming Common Problems

Coping with Rheumatism and Arthritis

DR KEITH SOUTER

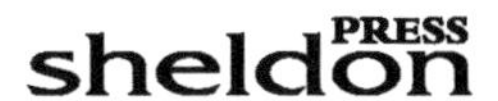

First published in Great Britain in 2010

Sheldon Press
36 Causton Street
London SW1P 4ST
www.sheldonpress.co.uk

British Library Cataloguing-in-Publication Data

A catalogue record for this book is available from the British Library

ISBN 978–1–84709–093–5

1 3 5 7 9 10 8 6 4 2

Typeset by Fakenham Photosetting Ltd, Fakenham, Norfolk
Printed in Great Britain by Ashford Colour Press

Produced on paper from sustainable forests

For my mother-in-law, Kathleen Kitchen, who has never allowed arthritis to get in the way of her enjoyment of life – an inspiration to us all

'The best medicine that I know for rheumatism is to thank the Lord that it ain't gout.'

Josh Billings, American humourist, 1818–1885

Contents

Acknowledgements

This book is the fruit of many years of medical practice. It is offered as an aid to anyone who has a rheumatic or arthritic condition in the hope that it will contribute to the way in which they deal with their health.

I have several people to thank for their help in writing this book. First of all, Isabel Atherton, my wonderful agent at Creative Authors, who initiated the process and whose help and encouragement at every stage of the book has been a delight.

Fiona Marshall, the commissioning editor at Sheldon Press, actually gave me the germ of the idea for the book and I am grateful to her. Then I must thank Robert Whittle, who copy-edited the manuscript and made several valuable suggestions which improved the readability of the text. And I thank Sally Green for bringing the various strands together to produce this finished volume.

And of course I must thank my patients, past and present, who in different ways have helped me to develop some of the ideas in this book. I hope that it will be of help to others.

Introduction

The number of people in the UK troubled by rheumatism and arthritis seems to be increasing year by year. About 20 per cent of all GP consultations are for these and related musculoskeletal conditions, making this the largest group of patients attending surgeries up and down the country. Although these disorders are not in themselves a major cause of death, they are the largest cause of pain and disability. Over three million adults are physically disabled because of such problems.

As we shall see in the following chapters, arthritis and rheumatism are blanket terms that cover a great many different conditions. Osteoarthritis is the most common form of arthritis, currently affecting more than eight million people in the UK. In addition, there are about a million people with rheumatoid arthritis. And people of all ages can be affected by these conditions. For example, some 15,000 children have juvenile arthritis. Fibromyalgia syndrome is a soft tissue condition that is being increasingly recognized as a significant problem. It is even more common than rheumatoid arthritis.

There are, of course, many excellent treatments available through the NHS, including a whole array of drugs, physiotherapy and even surgery. All of these have their place and as a doctor I have used them all in my management of patients with many of these rheumatic conditions. Yet it has to be said that they also have their limitations and there is much that can be achieved through self-help. Indeed, it is my experience after 30 years as a GP that people cope with their condition best when they are actively involved in its management, rather than just being the passive recipient of a drug or other treatment. I firmly believe that self-help is fundamental to coping with and managing these conditions, and I want to introduce you to a way of thinking that will help you to apply some very effective self-help methods.

In this book, I take an unashamedly pragmatic approach, as I have done throughout my career. Whenever I have found that something has helped patients, I have explored it and often incorporated it into my armamentarium of things to offer others to deal with their problem. I include here orthodox and complementary methods and even some that have been derived from my studies into folk medicine.

After qualifying as a GP, I trained in acupuncture and later obtained specialist accreditation in homoeopathic medicine with the Faculty of Homoeopathy. In addition, for many years I also used hypnotherapy and relaxation techniques in my practice. Nutrition has always been of fundamental importance to me and time and time again I have found that simply modifying a person's diet can transform his or her life. It is my impression that almost 50 per cent of people will benefit to some degree through nutritional means.

But the greatest potential weapon that all people have is their mind and their insight into themselves. This is one of the main concepts that I want to get across in this book, for there really is a great deal that you can do to help yourself as long as you get your mind working for you. That means taking control, refusing to allow negativity to let you feel isolated or fall into the idea that you are a sufferer. You must transform yourself into someone who copes with and manages a condition. There really is no need to think that you are doomed to a downward spiral of increasing pain and disability.

Note This book is not intended to replace advice from your doctor. Do consult your doctor if you are experiencing symptoms with which you feel you need help.

1

Self-awareness and self-help – the most important chapter in the book

Life will always be to a large extent what we ourselves make it.

Self-Help, Dr Samuel Smiles, 1859[1]

When I first qualified as a doctor I had a rather naive belief that medicine and surgery could solve most health problems. After all, we had wonderful drugs that could suppress all sorts of symptoms, kill off a vast array of microbes, top up the body's hormones or modify disease processes. Medical research was gradually pushing back the frontiers of knowledge and surgical techniques were advancing in an almost exponential manner. It did not take long in medical practice, however, to realize that this was a false belief.

This is not to say that modern medicine and surgery do not have amazing successes, for clearly they do. As a practitioner I have prescribed all the orthodox treatments over a 30-year period. Yet it has to be said that sometimes, despite being given the best available treatments, people do still struggle with their health. This particularly seems to be the case with rheumatic and arthritic conditions. Yet as I discovered, there is a vast amount that the individual can do in terms of self-help.

Please note that I am not suggesting a method to be used instead of your orthodox treatment. What I am putting before you is a means of looking at how your medical condition is affecting you throughout the many levels of your life. If you consider the logic of this you will see how different strategies can be mobilized to manage your condition better. This may mean that you will be able to take fewer pain-killers, get more mobility and enjoy life more than you have been doing.

The germ of an idea

I said in the introduction that I have taken a pragmatic approach in this book, just as I have done in my medical practice over 30 years. By this I mean that as a doctor I have taken the opportunity to learn from my patients even as I have been treating them. Where I have seen benefits and improvements from things that I have administered or that they have independently been using, I have explored and investigated. And where there have been clear benefits from some method or snippet of advice, I have incorporated it into my range of treatment options to pass on to others. That actually seems to be the way that many doctors practise. They develop their pattern of practice heuristically, or by experience of seeing what helps and what does not.

As I went about my daily work it became clear to me, however, that 'one hat will not fit all heads'. In other words, not everyone with one condition will respond to one type of treatment. That is a truism in all branches of medicine. So what could one do to become more effective? One thing that dawned upon me was that just as every person was unique, coming to the consultation with his or her own personality, needs and agenda, so did I present a different face to each person. By this I mean that after a few moments general chat at the start of the consultation, I became quite adept at gauging the sort of approach the patient was looking for. For example, did he or she want a solid diagnosis and my best scientific explanation, or to explore his or her feelings about a particular problem, or to consider some alternative manner of dealing with the problem? I realized that in a sense I adopted a chameleon-like approach. Effectively, I tried to match my consultation style to that of the person and his or her individual needs. This, I have to confess, is the way that I consult, and it is the manner that I have found most effective. I found the unvarying 'here I am, this is what you get' approach to be limited and less effective.

I had entered general practice from psychiatry so I was very interested in the psychological aspect of medicine. In psychiatry I had learned the rudiments of hypnotherapy and relaxation techniques and I maintained my interest by incorporating these into my practice and attending various courses. I also studied various techniques from the fields of cognitive behavioural therapy (CBT), neuro-linguistic programming, (NLP) and various types of psychotherapy. There was an inescapable basic sense about them. And that very basic sense was to form the principle of my whole approach to medicine in general, but also to the self-help way of thinking, on which I expand later in this chapter.

Before I do this, permit me to lapse into a little anecdotage to explain some of the experiences and influences that have helped me arrive at this approach. I want to do this because for many people 'self-help' conjures up images of copper or magnetic bracelets, health shops and shelves full of various supplements, some special diet or another, or some form of complementary medicine. While these are all potential forms of self-help, to my mind there has to be something deeper than that, something more significant. To use my earlier example, these are just hats of different sizes, which may fit some but not all heads. I think that it is often necessary to broaden the search, and I would say that it is not just a question of which hat size is needed, but whether the person needs a hat, an overcoat, an umbrella or even gumboots!

An old bottle of embrocation

Not long after I started work as a GP I had a salutary experience. For several weeks I had been vainly struggling to help a patient with a back problem. I had tried all the accepted conventional treatments, but without any success whatsoever. I was surprised, therefore, to see him fairly march into my consulting room one morning. He grinned broadly as he stood to attention by the desk, and suddenly jack-knifed forward to touch his toes. Before I could check my notes to see which of my remedies had finally worked he whipped out a filthy-looking bottle from a pocket, uncorked it and wafted it under my nose.

It smelled awful. 'Deldoc!' he announced. 'A farmer friend of mine treats his animals with it. Works a treat. I just rub this on and the pains and stiffness go. I thought you should know about it.'

He was a much happier chap than he had been when I had been treating him and he left, taking his foul-smelling bottle with him. I suspected his case was illustrative of the placebo effect and although he had marched off, I thought I would see him again fairly soon. The placebo effect, as we had been taught in medical school, is generally thought to be fairly short in action (and we shall look at this soon).

Yet he didn't come back and I saw him about town as well as on the local golf course. It set me thinking about this 'deldoc' of his. I needed to know more about it so I went to the library to track it down. But I could find no mention of it anywhere. Chance played a hand and I came across a reference while I was reading a book on the history of medicine. But this was not a reference to 'deldoc,' but to 'opodeldoc', a camphorated soap liniment, usually fortified with various herbs and oils, which had been devised by Paracelsus[2] in the sixteenth century.

A few weeks after this I was fortunate enough to meet my patient's farmer friend. I told him that I was fascinated by folk medicine and by his embrocation, which had worked so well for his friend. I asked him about what he used if his 'deldoc' failed.

'Hurtication,' he replied, in a fine Yorkshire accent. He outlined his method of harvesting fresh nettles and flailing the painful part and surrounding area. One could see why it would work, for it would be bound to hurt. This counter-irritation would over-ride the original pain.

After some thought, however, it dawned on me that perhaps this remedy might also have undergone a name change over the years. I thought it likely that this time, instead of losing a letter, it may have gained one to produce a plausible sounding word. Thus, for 'hurtication' read 'urtication'.

Urtication, from the Latin *urtica* for nettle, is a technique of considerable antiquity. In one form it was used by the Romans for the treatment of rheumatic conditions, and in mediaeval times it was used as a treatment for bed-wetting.

I found this fascinating, for several reasons. First, it added to an idea that I had been mulling over for some time – of a vast pool of folk medicine that people tap into – and second, methods that were once part of accepted practice were jettisoned, yet somehow seeped into that folk medicine pool. Opodeldoc had resurfaced in my consulting room after several hundred years.

Cider vinegar and honey

At about the same time, I came across an interesting book entitled *Folk Medicine*, first published in 1958 by a family physician, Dr DeForrest C. Jarvis. So successful was it that he followed it up in 1960 with *Arthritis and Folk Medicine*. Apparently, he had written this second book in response to the countless letters he received from readers of *Folk Medicine*, asking for his advice about methods to deal with their arthritis.

Dr Jarvis was a fifth generation native of Vermont in the USA. He was born in 1881 and started in medical practice in 1909. He was rural medicine editor of *Medical World* and a member of the American Academy of Otolaryngology and Ophthalmology. He lived and practised family medicine for 50 years among the tough hard-working mountain folk of the state of Vermont. Over the years he studied the folk medicine that they used to help themselves, and where he found that it had helped, he incorporated it into his practice. In particular he looked at nutrition and remedies that could be used to both treat and fend off such problems as chronic fatigue, excessive catarrh, bowel spasms, and rheumatism and arthritis. He advocated the use of kelp, iodine, castor oil, corn oil, honey and cider vinegar.

I liked his approach. He was a good observer and he believed that there was much that could be learned from nature. And so he quietly and methodically went about observing bees, birds, wild animals and farm animals. He talked to farmers about how they managed the health and ailments of their animals, and at the same time he observed his patients and their responses to his dietary manipulation. In addition, he watched the effects of weather on people, especially those who suffered from arthritis. He wrote about all this in a clear and simple style.

Dr Jarvis was very interested in his patients' dietary habits and came to the conclusion, mainly through empirical observation and good logic, that there was no such thing as an ideal diet. People are individuals and it is a question of getting them on the diet that is going to be right for them. This certainly struck a chord with me.

He also defined what he called 'the three Rs of folk medicine.' These were Resistance, Repair and Recovery. Impair any one of them and you have a health problem. And he searched for ways that he could improve all of them.

In addition to dietary advice, Dr Jarvis advocated the use of whole cider vinegar and unpasteurized honey, which became formulated as 'Honegar'. It was not long before I became aware that many of my patients were in fact using honey and apple cider vinegar in the self-treatment of their rheumatic disorders. And many of them swore by it!

Dr Jarvis was of the opinion that this worked in arthritis and rheumatism because people did not take enough acid into their system. The acidity of the apple cider vinegar, buffered by the natural healing power of honey, would in his opinion restore the body's balance.

Interestingly, in the early 1980s, Margaret Hills, a registered nurse in the UK, cured herself from debilitating arthritis by using the regimen advocated in Dr Jarvis's book. Later she opened a clinic herself specializing in the treatment of arthritis using cider vinegar, honey and crude black molasses, together with a regime of Epsom salts baths. In 1985 she wrote a book, *Curing Arthritis the Drug-Free Way* (Sheldon Press), outlining her method. This became a bestseller and was followed by several others.

Sister Hills's concept was different from that of Dr Jarvis. She was of the opinion that arthritis and rheumatism was caused by excess acid in the system as a result of eating too much acid-producing food. There is a paradox between these two authors, for both advocated cider vinegar. Nonetheless, many people did seem to find it of benefit.

The misunderstood placebo effect

I mentioned the placebo effect in my first little anecdote. I think it is important to discuss it before we move on. Essentially, it is the effect by which an ineffective drug or treatment somehow makes someone feel better. The word comes from the Latin *placere*, meaning 'to please'.

Scientists regard the placebo effect as a bit of a nuisance in research. Yet it is, in my opinion, a fascinating phenomenon, possibly the most fascinating phenomenon in the whole of medicine. For some reason (possibly for many reasons) a person may respond to an inactive agent in a very positive manner. Nowadays placebos are used in scientific trials, usually double-blind trials, in which neither the patient nor the doctor knows whether they are being given an active agent or a placebo. This sort of trial is used to assess whether a drug (the active agent) is superior to the placebo – in other words, better than nothing. This is called an explanatory trial, in which the researchers are trying to determine if the treatment actually has a specific effect.[3]

The problem is that a placebo response can occur in anything from between 25 and 70 per cent of cases. The most frequently reported placebo response is 30 per cent, but it depends upon many factors. In general, the more dramatic the treatment, the greater the placebo response. Surgery, being the most dramatic type of treatment should, therefore, have the highest placebo response.

In studies on medicines, it has been found that red, yellow or brown tablets or capsules work best, whereas green and blue work less well. It has also been found that the smaller the tablets or pills the better.

In days gone by placebos were prescribed liberally. In 1905, Sir William Osler, the doyen of early twentieth-century physicians said that 'man has an inborn desire to take medicine; it is one of the things that separates him from the animals.' Implicit in this was the suggestion that man also responds to the idea of taking a medicine.

Nowadays it is considered unethical to use placebos in a therapeutic setting, their use being purely reserved for clinical trials. I agree with this wholeheartedly, yet I do not consider the *placebo effect* to be a nuisance. It is something that happens in all therapeutic situations and it cannot and need not be removed. People may dismiss a benefit as being 'all in the mind'. To this I would ask, what is the matter with that? As we shall see later in Chapter 5, on pain, the emotions are intimately involved in the perception of chronic pain. The emotions also affect how one thinks, so if you can modify them, this can only be a good thing. Getting the patient's mind to work is always one of my aims.

In short, I believe that the placebo effect means that for some reason the individual is exhibiting a degree of self-healing. And that is what we want to happen. The placebo is misunderstood and, rather than being written off as a statistical nuisance in research, it should be the subject of intense study. It may hold the key to self-healing.

In this book I am not advocating the taking of placebos or of doing anything that is known to be ineffective. As I say, I favour a pragmatic approach and if it works, try it. Some of the things may work for you, others may not. This you will find out for yourself.

The lesson I learned

From what I have just said about the placebo effect, what do you make of the examples I gave of opodeldoc, cider vinegar and honey? Do you think any beneficial effect would be real, or would it be entirely due to a placebo effect? Or doesn't it matter?

Well, my own view is that the opodeldoc could have a short-term real effect, for it is a rubefacient. There are many of these available over the counter, or on prescription from your doctor. This word comes from the Latin *rubor*, meaning redness. Effectively, it depends upon the compounds it contains producing a dilatation of the blood vessels under the skin. Thus the area goes red, and it may feel hot and start to itch a bit. We call this 'counter-irritation', whereby you induce one pain, a different type of pain from the one that is causing the problem, to produce an 'over-ride' of the original pain. This is a legitimate method of treating pain, which is discussed in Chapter 5.

In the case of the cider vinegar and honey you will note that its two advocates, Dr D. C. Jarvis and Sister Margaret Hills, give conflicting reasons for its efficacy. Yet both reported that many thousands of people benefit from it. Yet, as you read more about their methods, you will find that the cider vinegar and honey are not the sole ingredients of their methods. They both advocated dietary and lifestyle change. This, I think, is significant.

I am not sure how cider vinegar and honey could really affect the highly efficient acid–base balance of the body, which automatically does all that it can to maintain the pH of the blood through several different mechanisms. So it could simply be the placebo effect. Or it could be a result of the dietary alteration and lifestyle change that was also being advocated. And yet again, it could be to do with the fact that because individuals are doing something for themselves, they are mentally taking charge of their health and doing something that they feel positive about. An improvement in the way that they feel could well be the result.

The conclusion I reached was that people fare best when they are actively involved in their own management, when they are content in other areas of their life besides their health, and most importantly when they feel that they can make effective changes that affect the quality of their life. This is taking a holistic or whole-person view. Good, effective self-help works best, in my opinion, if one develops a holistic way of thinking.

The life cycle

This heading of 'the life cycle' may take you back to biology lessons when you looked at the different life cycles of insects, fish, frogs and other creatures on the evolutionary ladder. I am not, however, using the term here in the same sense. I am using it as a model for a person's life. This has nothing to do with the person's development with age, but is to do with the different levels or spheres that make up one's life at any point in time. And you will see that there is a cycle involved, certainly in the manner in which a condition, virtually any chronic medical condition, can affect people.

Yet to use the biology analogy a little longer, you will learn a certain amount about fish by dissecting them to look at their internal organs. But you won't know how they move and feed without studying them in water. And you won't learn about their behaviour with other fish and predators unless you observe them in a realistic environment. Even then you will not get to know about them fully unless you just become a total observer of them.

So it is in medicine. In order to help people, you need to know as much as possible about their condition, their symptoms and the things that make their symptoms better or worse. And ideally you want to know about their habits, their diet, their desires, their fears, their relationships and so on. That might seem like a tall order, but if you can build up such a picture of a person, you can see how a condition is truly affecting that person throughout all levels of life.

And this is what *you* need to do in order to help yourself manage a condition in the most effective way that you can. It is the aim of this book to show you.

There are five levels or spheres of life that we need to consider:

1 Body – what symptoms you have (e.g. pain, stiffness, tiredness).
2 Emotions – how does it make you feel (e.g. anxious, sad, depressed, angry, jealous of others who are not affected).
3 Mind – how it affects the type of thoughts you have (e.g. pessimistic thoughts, negative thoughts, self-defeating thoughts).
4 Behaviour – how it makes you behave (e.g. isolating yourself by avoiding things or other people, developing habits such as smoking or drinking, becoming inactive).
5 Lifestyle – how it affects your ability to do things, your relationships, and also how events in your life impact on you.

Look at Figure 1.1. You will see the five spheres, starting with the body sphere at the top. If you follow it clockwise you will see that it follows

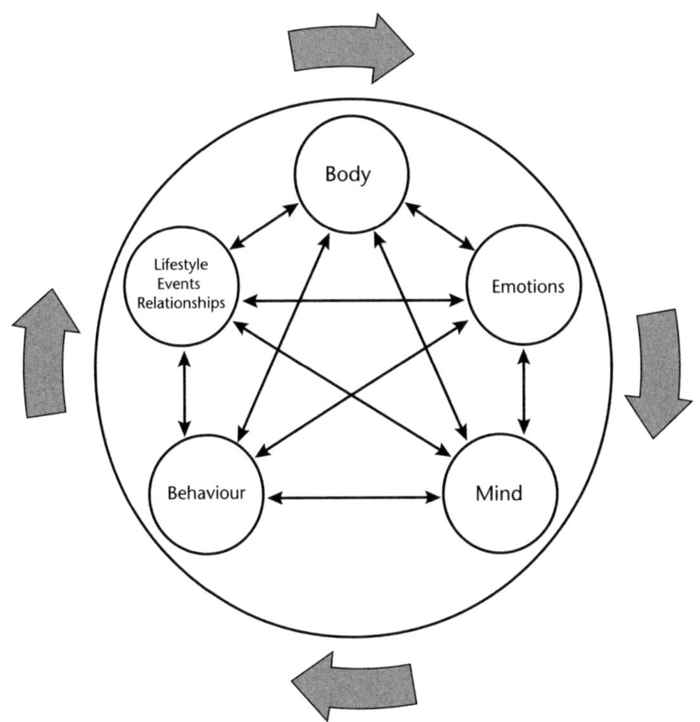

Figure 1.1 The five spheres of life and their interactions one to the other

the order above – body, emotions, mind, behaviour, lifestyle. And note the outer circle that encloses the whole structure. This represents the person's whole self, his or her life. In other words the five spheres all make up part of the person's experience of life.

Notice also that there are double-headed arrows between the spheres. The outer arrows represent the general progression, because the order represents the way that a condition will tend to have its impact on a person. The condition produces physical or body symptoms. If these persist for a while they tend to affect the person emotionally. You will start to feel something about the symptoms or about the condition. The emotions make you think in a particular way. The condition may come to dominate your thoughts: you worry about how it will progress, how it is going to impact on your wellbeing, your work, your family. This can affect your behaviour in that you may stop doing certain things or you may take up various habits. And this may affect your lifestyle and your relationships. And again, this may intensify the condition at the physical level.

Notice also the inner double-headed arrows – they represent the ways that the different spheres are affected by the other spheres. Indeed, each sphere is potentially affected by all the others.

I am sure that you will see that a physical condition has the potential to affect all the spheres or levels of your life. This is very important, because the double-headed arrows also indicate that you have multiple potential ways in which you can affect a physical condition.

Ronald

Ronald is a 39-year-old postal worker who developed psoriatic arthropathy (see Chapter 3). He had been troubled with psoriasis on his skin for 12 years, but over six months he had started to experience painful swelling and stiffness in his hands and his knees. He had become disabled very quickly and had quite correctly been referred by his GP for a specialist rheumatological opinion. This ultimately resulted in him being treated with a drug called methotrexate.

His skin had always been a nuisance, but the arthropathy really took its toll. It stopped him playing golf and stopped him working and it began to have an impact on his home life. He started to feel depressed and anxious about the future. Because of this he became very negative, pessimistic and irritable. He became resentful of people who seemed fitter than himself yet who did not take as much care of their health as he had done. He stopped going out, started to drink more frequently, ate a lot of junk food and picked arguments with his family members. His symptoms proved difficult to control despite his medication.

And you can see just how his condition had an impact on him, as a progression around the spheres. Effectively his life cycle was operative and he was chained into the condition, which manifested its effect throughout his whole life.

In going through the life cycle, Ronald was able to see that the spheres of body, emotions and behaviour stood out for him and that they had had an impact on the others. In other words, he was able to identify the interaction of these spheres, so that he could start to do something about it. He was also aware that his family would prefer a dad who didn't drink and who was less angry. His dominant emotions were anger and guilt. He felt guilty because he felt that he was failing his family.

There is no need to go further than that. I hope that you will see how this life cycle concept can help you to identify potential ways for you to self-help.

Self-awareness

According to the ancient Greek writer Pausanius, the aphorism 'Know thyself' was inscribed in the forecourt of the Temple of Apollo at Delphi. This was where people would come to consult the famous Delphic Oracle. This is a piece of wisdom that most people would do well to consider.

If you have absorbed the basic concept of the life cycle you have already made a start. Yet there is more that is worth considering. Do you, for instance have a low or a high pain threshold? Do you have an optimistic or a pessimistic outlook? Are you an angry person, or are you placid? Are you a hurried person, or are you laid-back? Are you assertive or submissive? Do you hold grudges or do you let things go? Are you a perfectionist or are you sloppy? Are you a victim?

There are many things worth knowing about yourself, because they can all have a bearing on how a condition can affect you. You may not feel that you relate to any of the above, or you may be somewhere in between on some. And they may have a part to play in how arthritis and rheumatism can affect you, although not necessarily in the way that you think.

Self-awareness is an important tool in your self-help kit. As we will see, it is worth taking an honest look at yourself. It is not always easy, but it may pay dividends.

Start using the life cycle straight away

That is right. I mean straight away. Get a fresh exercise book and on the first page draw the life cycle. Familiarize yourself with it so that it becomes second nature to you. Think about each of the spheres and how they relate to your life. Allocate two facing pages to each of them in sequence. You can use the left side for negative pieces of information and the right page for the positives. Start by putting one major piece of information on each page. On the positive page think of things that may bring relief, such as listening to music. You may find that they all relate to a particular symptom or they may not. But they are all important, since they affect your life. And since all these spheres are inter-related, by being able to modify any one of them you will affect others.

For example, under 'Body' you might put pain, stiffness, tiredness or any other symptom that you experience. Under 'Emotions' you might put anxiety, anger, guilt and so on. And under 'Lifestyle' you might put relationship difficulty, financial difficulties, sexual problem, dangerous occupation, troublesome boss or whatever is relevant.

Spend time mulling it over. You may find some spheres are almost empty, although I suspect not. You will start to see a pattern developing. And you will start to see interactions. And you will almost certainly see that these interactions open up potential to do something about your life and the way that your arthritis or rheumatic condition is affecting you.

Think again about Ronald's case, above. His perception was that his spheres of body, emotions and behaviour were the problem ones. He actually drew his life cycle with those spheres much larger than the others. But it was the interacting arrows that he found most useful, since he realized that by working on his behaviour he could improve his emotions so that he was better able to manage his physical symptoms.

If you are a visual type of person (like Ronald), you might find that re-drawing your life cycle to show the relevant sizes of the spheres gives you an idea of the shape of your life (and remember the outer circle, which represents your life). You may see that it bulges in particular parts of the life cycle. Your aim is to re-balance it all.

On the other hand if you are a more number-oriented person, you might try scoring these things. Work out a score out of 10 (or 20 or even 100) for each sphere and write those scores down in the spheres. However you can get the idea of the way the spheres distort your life, that is the best way for you.

The essence of it is that you will see what areas of your life you feel you are going to need to address.

We shall be looking at this as we go, but once you have done this, you have made a good start on your way to self-help.

2

The locomotor system

The locomotor system is the collective name given to the bones, joints and muscles that we use to move about (Figure 2.1). Before I start talking about rheumatism and arthritis it is important to have some understanding of the locomotor system so that you can understand how the various rheumatic conditions can cause problems.

Bones

Some bones in the skeleton are protective, such as the bones of the skull, the pelvis and the ribcage, whereas others are structural and involved mainly in the business of locomotion. When you were born you would have had over 300 bones of assorted size. As you grow up many of these fuse together so that you end up as an adult with 206.

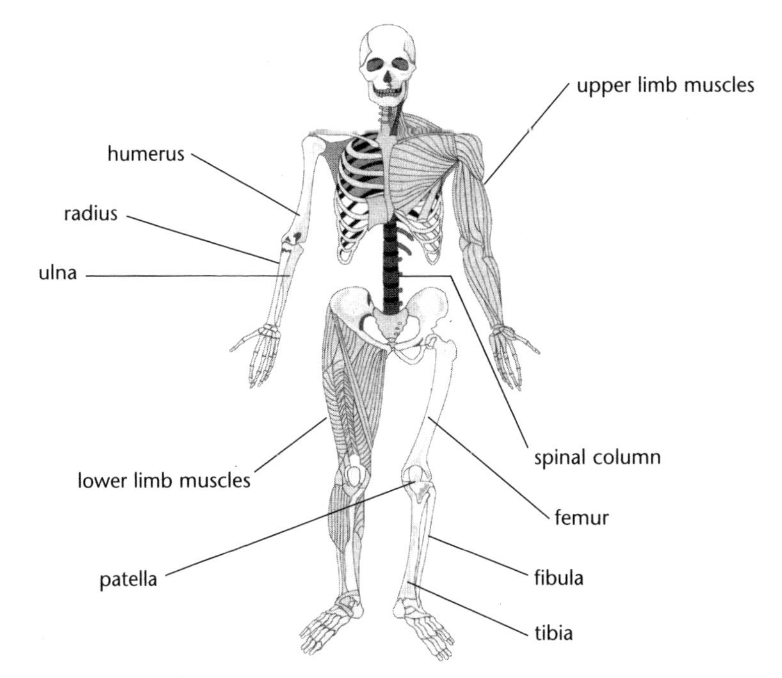

Figure 2.1 The locomotor system

Latin is the language of anatomy and all the bones have Latin names. They might sound strange, but the meanings are often quite instructive, informative and even poetic. Let us look at a few.

The *femur* or thigh bone means exactly that, the thigh. It is the largest bone in the body, and the strongest. Its rounded head fits into the socket end of the pelvis to form the largest ball-and-socket joint in the body. This socket is called the *acetabulum*, meaning 'vinegar cup' or 'cruet'. The name goes back to the days of Pliny the Elder,[4] who wrote about its similarity to a vinegar cruet.

The two shin bones are called the *tibia* and the *fibula*. The tibia is the largest one and means 'flute.' It was called this because in Roman times musicians used the tibias of animals and birds to make flutes and pipes. The fibula, the smaller bone on the outer shin, means 'brooch-pin', and indeed, beside the tibia it looks like a brooch-fastener.

The name for the kneecap is the *patella*, which means 'saucer'. It sits like an upside-down saucer on the front of the kneecap. It is also interesting because it is an unusual type of bone called a sesamoid bone. This term was first used by the ancient Greek physician Galen[5] in the second century AD, because he thought that they resembled sesame seeds. Such bones form within certain tendons where they rub on convex body surfaces. The patella is the largest sesamoid bone in the body.

The *humerus* is the bone of the upper arm. The two forearm bones were also named in antiquity. The *ulna* is the larger of the two and means 'elbow'. Its pointed end at the elbow is called the *olecranon*, and it is a common site of a type of bursitis (see Chapter 4). The other forearm bone is the *radius*, which means 'spoke'. It was given this name by Galen because of its resemblance to the spoke of a chariot's wheel.

The bones are made up of living tissue. The bone cells are continually at work, involved in the growth and repair of your skeleton. Some of the bones are hollow and contain bone marrow, needed to manufacture your red and white blood cells.

Cartilage

Cartilage is a very important type of connective tissue. It is made up of cells called chondrocytes. These cells produce an extracellular matrix composed of complex substances called glycoproteins, collagen and elastic fibres. It has no nerve supply and no direct blood supply so it has to derive nutrients by diffusion from surrounding body fluids and tissue.

There are three types of cartilage:

- Hyaline cartilage is hard and is found in the nose, the larynx and covering the bones in synovial joints.
- Elastic cartilage is very flexible and is found in the ear.
- Fibrocartilage is tough but with some flexibility. It is found in the intervertebral discs of the spine, in the symphysis pubis, the joint at the very front of the pelvis and at the attachment of certain ligaments and tendons.

The cartilage that covers the ends of bones is 65–85 per cent water, and there is a tendency for it to lose fluid and dry out as one ages. Degeneration of this cartilage is very important in arthritic conditions. Incredibly, it is about eight times more slippery than ice.

Joints

Our joints allow us to move freely and dexterously. You may be surprised to know that you have 230 of these moveable and flexible joints in the body. Essentially, a joint is any part in the body where two bones meet. They can be classified either according to structure or function.

A structural classification of joints:

- Fibrous joints, where the bones are connected by fibrous connective tissue.
- Cartilaginous joints, where the bones are connected by cartilage.
- Synovial joints, where the bones do not actually meet, but are enclosed in a capsule containing synovial fluid.

A functional classification of joints:

- Synarthrodial joints, which have virtually no movement – most of these are fibrous joints, such as the bones of the skull.
- Amphiarthrodial joints, which have slight movement – most of these are cartilaginous joints, such as those found in the pelvis and between the vertebrae that make up the spine.
- Synovial joints, which have a lot of movement; there are several types, and these are the most important joints for us to consider, since they are the ones most likely to be affected by arthritis.

As you can see, the two classifications virtually match.

Synovial joints

Synovial joints are by far the most common joints in the body. They are characterized by being surrounded by an articular capsule, which has a special lining called the synovial membrane. This membrane

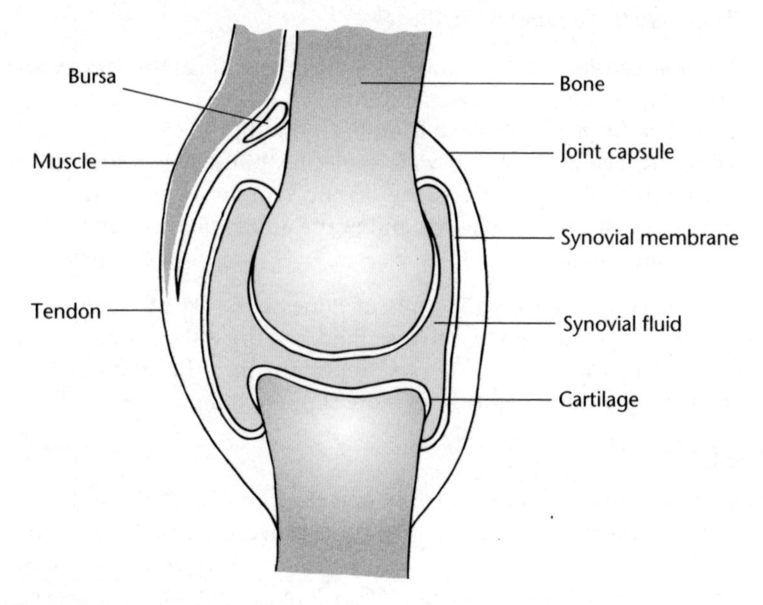

Figure 2.2 A synovial joint

produces synovial fluid, which lubricates the joints and supplies nutrients to the cartilage; it also contains cells that mop up any debris or microbes that manage to get into the joint. The bone ends are covered in cartilage, which acts as a shock absorber and as a gliding surface. Most synovial joints have ligaments inside or outside the capsule, which both support the joint and limit its movements (Figure 2.2).

Significantly, synovial fluid is a thixotropic fluid, which means that it can vary in its viscosity. This can be one of the causes of stiffness in rheumatic disorders (see Chapter 6).

Synovial joints are located predominantly in limbs, and because of the large range of movements of these joints, they can be shoved out of place or dislocated when they are injured.

The movement of these joints is determined by their anatomical shape, the size of the capsule and hence the amount of distance between the bones, and by the muscles, tendons and ligaments that surround them.

Bursae (singular, bursa, from the Latin for 'purse' or 'wine-skin') are flat sacs containing synovial fluid. They are found around all the major synovial joints. These allow muscles and other tissues to glide smoothly over them and cushion them from the underlying bone.

There are six types of synovial joint:

1 Ball-and-socket joints, such as the hip and shoulder joints. These joints are the most mobile of all the joints. They permit you to swing your arms and legs in many different directions.
2 Hinge joints, such as at the knee and elbow. These joints allow movement in one direction, rather like the opening and closing of a hinged door.
3 Ellipsoidal joints, such as the joint at the base of your index finger, or between the radius and the scaphoid bone at the wrist. These joints are formed by an egg-shaped bone-end fitting into a concave cavity of the same shape. As such they allow bending and extending, and rocking from side to side. They are similar to ball-and-socket joints, but the magnitude of their movement is less.
4 Gliding joints, which occur between the surfaces of two flat bones that are held together by ligaments. Some of the wrist and ankle bones move by gliding against each other.
5 Pivot joints, such as the pivot joint between the atlas and the axis, the two top bones in your neck. These joints only allow rotation, as when you turn your head from side to side.
6 Saddle joints, such as in your thumbs. These joints are rather like a saddle on a horse's back. The bones in a saddle joint can rock back and forth and from side to side, but they have limited rotation.

From this brief run through of the joints you can see how they are adapted for the different types of movement that is needed. The skull bones don't need to move because they provide protection to the brain. The pelvic joints don't need to move much at all (except during pregnancy and labour in women). Hinge joints like the knees need to move only in one direction, whereas ball-and-socket joints like the hips and the shoulder need to be rotational. And those precious thumbs benefit from having those curious saddle joints. You can get an idea of the way that a condition may limit the action of a joint. Now we finish this chapter with a consideration of the all-important tissues that enable us to move our joints.

The soft tissues

The soft tissues are the tissues and structures that move the joints – the muscles, tendons and ligaments.

Muscles

There are over 650 muscles in the body and they are of three types – skeletal muscles, cardiac (heart) muscle, and smooth (visceral) muscles. We are only concerned here with the skeletal muscles. These are arranged in groups around the joints, their function being to move the joints. They account for between 40 and 50 per cent of the body weight.

Most muscles have a similar structure, consisting of a fleshy contractile part known as the muscle belly, a point of origin and a point of insertion. The point of origin is where the muscle is anchored to bone. The point of insertion is where it is attached to the bone that it has the job of moving.

Muscles are arranged in opposing pairs. Each muscle is capable of pulling in only one direction. The muscle that it is paired with pulls in the opposite direction. When a muscle belly contracts it pulls the bone, at the point of insertion, towards it. At the same time the opposing muscle of the pair will relax. This is easiest understood by thinking of the biceps and the triceps muscles in the arm. When the biceps contracts it pulls the arm up towards the shoulder. When the triceps contracts it pulls in the opposite direction to straighten the arm.

We shall consider muscle structure in Chapter 6, on stiffness.

Tendons

A tendon (or sinew) is a tough band of fibrous connective tissue that connects the muscle to the bone. Tendons are made up of collagen. Some tendons, such as the fine ones in the hands, run in lubricated synovial sheaths.

Ligaments

Ligaments are small tough bands of tissue that connect the ends of bones together to form joints. They have a supporting and buffering function. They also limit the movements of joints.

3

Arthritis

As noted in the Introduction, the terms 'arthritis' and 'rheumatism' are both rather vague, consisting as they do of some 200 conditions. Arthritis essentially relates to those conditions that affect the joints. Rheumatism is a much more nebulous label, which includes those non-joint (non-articular) conditions that affect the soft tissues and supportive structures of the locomotor system.

This chapter considers the main types of arthritis – conditions that affect the joints. Chapter 4 looks at the main types of rheumatism, or non-joint rheumatic conditions.

Going to your doctor

It is very important to have a formal diagnosis made, so if joint problems are bothering you, such as pain, stiffness and tiredness, you should pay a visit to your doctor. The diagnosis may be very straightforward from the history that you give and from a simple physical examination. Your doctor will want to know about your symptoms and the way these interfere with your life. He may also consider any relevant family history, the presence of other conditions like psoriasis or colitis, any history of injury to joints or of any recent infections.

Often a diagnosis will not be possible just on the basis of the history and examination, in which case some basic tests will be asked for. These may include one or more of the following.

Blood tests

Full blood count

A full blood count (FBC) measures the numbers of all the different types of blood cells. An excess number of white cells could be indicative of an underlying infection. A deficiency of haemoglobin could point to the presence of anaemia, which is common in rheumatoid arthritis.

Erythrocyte sedimentation rate

The erythrocyte sedimentation rate (ESR) gives a fairly crude idea about the degree of stickiness of the blood cells and the presence of inflammation in the body. It does not in itself tell where this inflammation could be, but is useful in that it indicates that further investigation is merited. The ESR would be normal in osteoarthritis, which is the type of arthritis associated with 'wear and tear'. This is in contrast to rheumatoid arthritis, the inflammatory type, in which the ESR would be raised.

Rheumatoid factor

Rheumatoid factor (RF) is a specific type of antibody that is found in high levels in some people with rheumatoid arthritis. If it is slightly raised, it is not diagnostic of rheumatoid arthritis, but it could indicate that there is an increased risk of joint problems later on in life.

Antinuclear antibodies

Antinuclear antibodies are active against the cell nucleus. They are almost a mistake in that an auto-immune reaction has been set off, in which antibodies attack the body's own tissues or cells. They can be indicative of different types of inflammatory arthritis.

Uric acid

The level of uric acid is high in patients with gout.

X-rays

X-rays may be indicated, but they are not always useful. Most people over the age of 50 have some degree of osteoarthritis, but the correlation between the presence of bony outgrowths and symptoms of osteoarthritis is not reliable. Of more significance is reduction of joint space, which implies that the cartilage is being worn down, since cartilage is invisible on X-ray.

Erosions are also very significant. These are small holes in the bones in the joint itself. They are a feature of rheumatoid arthritis and other inflammatory types of arthritis, but not of osteoarthritis. These are seen on X-ray as small holes.

Bony outgrowths, known as osteophytes, are a characteristic X-ray feature of osteoarthritis. These are common in the neck and the lumbar spine or along joint margins.

Scans

The usual X-rays may not always help, and sometimes a 'deeper', more sophisticated investigation is needed. These will give a three-dimensional image.

Computerized tomography scans

Computerized tomography (CT) scans are essentially a composite of lots of X-rays taken from different angles to build up a three-dimensional image. A CT scan will thus give an impression of the structure of a joint, but not tell much about the soft tissues.

Magnetic resonance imaging scans

Magnetic resonance imaging (MRI) scanning is a very sophisticated investigation that uses magnetism, ultrasound and computerized technology to build up multiple images of the inside of the body. MRI scans may show changes in joints that do not show up on X-rays, and they can be useful in the early stages of rheumatoid arthritis. They also show up soft tissues. It can be an alarming investigation for people who are prone to claustrophobia, since sometimes it necessitates being advanced through a large tunnel-like apparatus.

Isotope bone scans

Sometimes it is necessary to give a small radiaoactive injection to allow the bones themselves to be imaged in order to see how well the bone cells (osteoblasts) are working. The amount of radioactivity is small. It is important to tell the nuclear imaging department if you are pregnant or breast-feeding.

DEXA scans

A DEXA or DXA (dual energy X-ray absorptiometry) scan is a bone densitometry scan, done on the lower spine and the hips and sometimes on the wrist as well, in order to determine the density of the bones. A low bone density is seen in osteoporosis or can suggest a risk of developing osteoporosis.

Osteoarthritis – non-inflammatory arthritis

Osteoarthritis is by far the commonest type of arthritis. It has up until recently been regarded as a simple 'wear-and-tear' type of degenerative arthritis, almost a natural part of the ageing process. Inflammation is not usually found and the blood tests are usually normal. Nowadays, however, it is considered to be a disorder of the cartilage, caused by excessive activity of the chondrocytes in the cartilage tissue. As a result the cartilage dries out, loses its slipperiness, gets thinner and eventually cracks. The underlying bone seems to develop little outgrowths – osteophytes – that alter the shape and function of the joint and may end up producing joint deformity. Small bone cysts can develop, the bones can get hardened or thickened and on X-ray you can see cracks or micro-fractures. At the moment we do not know what starts this process.

As mentioned earlier, most people over 50 would show some degree of osteoarthritic changes if they were to have an X-ray. In fact, about 80 per cent have these changes, but only a quarter of them will have pain. Men are more likely to have osteoarthritic problems under 45, but after 55 women are more likely to be affected.

Osteoarthritis most commonly affects the cervical spine (the neck), the lumbar spine (the lower back), the hips, the knees and the hands. In total, more than eight million people in the UK are affected. Of this number, six million have painful osteoarthritis of one or both knees. About two million have some osteoarthritis of the hips, and about 650,000 have pain from their hips that necessitates treatment. Almost 60,000 hip replacements and about the same number of knee replacements are carried out in England and Wales each year, the majority being done because of osteoarthritis.

The main symptoms of osteoarthritis are pains in the joints with stiffness and limitation of movement. Often the joints will swell and they may become warm. A characteristic feature is the presence of both Heberden's nodes on the last joints of the fingers and Bouchard's nodes on the middle joints (Figure 3.1).

Treatment

There are several mainstays of orthodox treatment for osteoarthritis:

1 Exercise, in order to maintain strength, flexibility and suppleness of the muscles and soft tissues around the joints.
2 Weight control, to reduce excessive strain on joints.

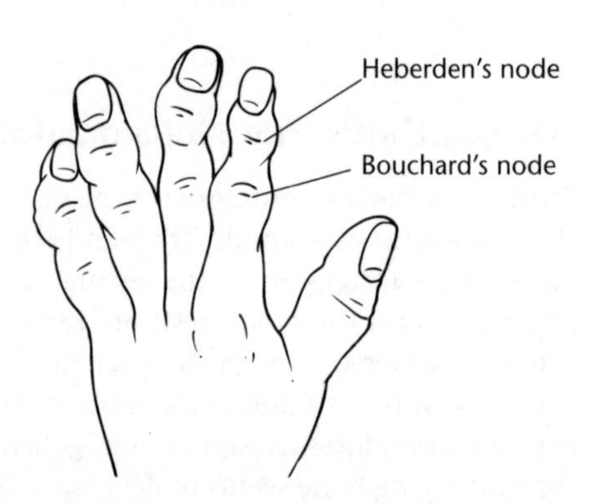

Figure 3.1 Characteristic changes in osteoarthritis of the hand

3 Joint protection, essentially to avoid further damage to joints.
4 Pain control, usually with pain-killers and sometimes anti-inflammatory drugs.

In addition, self-help is important. By using the life cycle approach you will see that there are many levels on which you can improve the way you view this condition. Surgery if necessary can transform a patient's life, yet even after there is much that self-help can do.

Secondary osteoarthritis

Secondary arthritis is exactly the same as osteoarthritis, except that it seems to arise from past injury or overuse of a particular joint. Accidents, much sporting activity in youth, repetitive strain and excessive weight can all play their part.

Rheumatoid arthritis

Rheumatoid arthritis is a completely different form of arthritis. Whereas osteoarthritis is not associated with inflammation, rheumatoid arthritis and most of the other types of arthritis are associated with a great deal of inflammation of the synovial joints.

There are currently about one million people with rheumatoid arthritis in the UK, with 26,000 new diagnoses a year. It is commoner in females than males, in a ratio of 3:1. Its peak age of onset is in the 30- to 50-year age band, although many youngsters under the age of 25 can also be affected.

Rheumatoid arthritis is a significant cause of disability. It is estimated that about 15 per cent of adults with rheumatoid arthritis will give up work within one year of diagnosis and that 40 per cent will have stopped working within five years, the majority as a result of their condition.

Rheumatoid arthritis is a complex condition that is actually a multi-system disorder. This means that it affects many of the systems of the body, not only the locomotor system. The blood, lungs, liver, kidney, skin and eyes can all be affected. It is an auto-immune condition, in that for some reason the body's immune system starts to produce antibodies that attack its own tissues. We do not know why this happens, although we are aware that some infections seem to trigger it off.

The main target of inflammation is the synovial membrane in the joints, the cartilage, the bursae and the tendon sheaths. The synovial membranes become thickened and, as a result, over-produce synovial

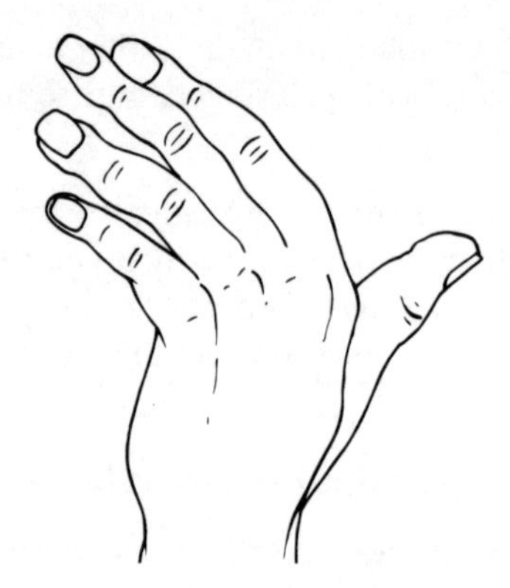

Figure 3.2 Characteristic changes in rheumatoid arthritis of the hand

fluid. They also seem to release other chemicals that produce further inflammation. The joints become swollen, and the cartilage and ligaments become damaged; so too does the underlying bone, and erosions appear in the bones.

Unlike osteoarthritis, rheumatoid arthritis tends to affect both sides of the body, and not just the large weight-bearing joints – it is more likely to affect the smaller and middle sized joints. Hence it attacks the fingers, wrists, elbows, knees, and ankles and feet. When the inflammation is very active the person may feel quite unwell, with fever, loss of appetite and sometimes marked weight loss.

The hands typically begin to show deformity of the joints, so that the fingers bend outwards, away from the thumbs and in the direction of the outer bone of the forearm, the ulna. This is termed ulnar deviation (Figure 3.2).

Stiffness and pain can be extremely hard to deal with. Early morning stiffness is one of the first features of the condition – it is hard and painful to move joints in the morning, but with some improvement as the day goes on.

Rheumatoid nodules are common. These nodules form as painless lumps at points under the skin where friction is common. Thus, they can form on the feet, ankles, backs of the hands and the elbows.

The eyes can be affected and become red and painful. Breathlessness can occur and various skin rashes can develop.

Rheumatoid arthritis is a condition that is subject to relapses and remissions. Active flare-ups or relapses are associated with increase in inflammation, when the joints can become more damaged.

When the blood is tested, the rheumatoid factor is likely to be high, there may be anaemia and some of the other inflammatory markers, such as the ESR, may be very high. There is a genetic marker called HLA-DR4, which is positive in 80 per cent of patients with rheumatoid arthritis.

Specialist referral

The nature of rheumatoid arthritis and its potential to damage joints and affect other systems are such that specialist referral is very important, and the earlier the better, since the aim of treatment is to control relapses with minimal joint damage and keep the person in remission for as long as possible.

In 2009 NICE (the National Institute for Clinical Excellence) modified its guidelines for the management of rheumatoid arthritis, and it now recommends that anyone with a persistent synovitis (inflamed synovial joint) of undetermined cause should be referred for a specialist opinion and management in a multi-disciplinary team. It also recommends that the referral should be urgent if the small joints of the hand or feet are affected.

Treatment

The aims of treatment are to:

- relieve symptoms;
- maintain function;
- protect joints;
- treat any problems in other systems of the body; and
- help the person to lead a normal life.

Many drugs are available to help, including pain-killers and non-steroidal anti-inflammatory drugs (NSAIDs). For many years these drugs were regarded as the first line of treatment for this condition. The problem is that, while they do reduce inflammation and ease pain, they do not have any effect on the long-term progression of the disease.

Disease-modifying anti-rheumatic drugs (DMARDs) is the name given to a whole cluster of drugs that may be used in rheumatoid arthritis. These are very powerful drugs, which have been shown to be capable of preventing joint damage and affecting the long-term progression of disease. They include the anti-malarial drugs hydroxychloroquine and chloroquine, gold, methotrexate, sulphasalazine, leflunamide, cyclosporine, cyclophosphamide and penicillamine. In addition to these drugs are the so-called biologics – etanercept, infliximab and adalimumab – which specifically affect the immune system.

In 2009 NICE also recommended that people with newly diagnosed active rheumatoid arthritis should be offered a combination of

DMARDs (including methotrexate and at least one other DMARD, plus a short course of corticosteroids) as a first line treatment as soon as possible, ideally within three months of the onset of persistent symptoms.

Scope for self-help with rheumatoid arthritis

I believe that there is always something that will help. I agree with the NICE recommendations and feel that the aim must be to modify the progression of the disease. The orthodox treatment is sensible and I would encourage people to go down this route. But I would also suggest looking at the life cycle approach and some of the measures that I cover in this book.

Sero-negative forms of arthritis

There are a number of other inflammatory arthritis conditions that have a superficial similarity to rheumatoid arthritis, but that do not cause a positive rheumatoid factor – hence they are referred to as the sero-negative arthropathies.

Ankylosing spondylitis

Ankylosing spondylitis is a chronic inflammatory condition of the spine, originally called Marie-Strumpell's disease or Bechterew's disease. It is a slowly progressive disorder that ultimately causes fusing of the vertebrae of the spinal column and the pelvis. When this occurs it produces a characteristic picture known as a 'bamboo spine' on X-ray. Males are more commonly affected than females, in a ratio of about 9:1. It usually starts in the 20s.

In some cases the peripheral joints are more affected to begin with, leading to a diagnosis of rheumatoid arthritis being made. The genetic marker HLA-B27 is positive in 95 per cent of patients with ankylosing spondylitis.

Anyone with suspected ankylosing spondylitis should be referred for specialist investigation and treatment. The aim of treatment is to maintain mobility, to try to avoid deformity and to control pain and inflammation.

Psoriatic arthropathy

Psoriatic arthropathy can also mimic rheumatoid arthritis, and occurs in people with psoriasis. The skin condition produces characteristic psoriatic lesions (although there are different types) and pitting of the nails. The arthropathy can affect the end joints of the fingers and toes and the knees.

If suspected, it is important to have a specialist opinion, since treatment with drugs like methotrexate can produce marked improvement in both the skin condition and the arthropathy.

Reactive arthritis

Reactive arthritis is a type of joint inflammation that affects one or more joints (usually symmetrically) and that occurs after an infection with various types of bacteria, viruses or other microbes, although the infection itself does not affect the joints. The infection can have been in the digestive tract as a gastroenteritis (e.g. with *Clostridium*, *Giardia* or *Campylobacter*, or in the urogenital tract, with *Chlamydia* or gonorrhoea). The genetic marker HLA-B27 can be positive in some patients. It is commonest in the 20- to 40-year age group, and is seen in males more than in females.

In some patients it can be associated with eye inflammation (conjunctivitis) and a urinary discharge (urethritis), in which case it is termed Reiter's syndrome.

When it occurs as reactive arthritis alone, the treatment usually consists of the prescription of anti-inflammatory agents and corticosteroid joint injections. It is usually followed by recovery after a few months.

Systemic lupus erythematosus

Systemic lupus erythematosus (SLE) is an auto-immune condition in which the immune system starts attacking various systems of the body, including the joints, the skin, the lungs, the kidneys and possibly the heart. It often produces profound fatigue. It is commoner in females than males in a ratio of 9:1. It usually affects women in their child-bearing years, from 15 to the mid-40s. It tends to have a waxing and waning nature with flare-ups of activity. It is not curable, but treatment can make it manageable.

One of the characteristic features is the presence of a butterfly red rash over the face. This is the description that you will find in all the textbooks, although when it was first described it was thought to give the person a wolf-like appearance, hence the name 'lupus'.

There is a milder variant called discoid lupus, in which the skin is the main target.

Scleroderma

Scleroderma is another auto-immune collagen disorder affecting the skin and the joints. The name comes from the Greek and means 'hard skin.' Effectively, the body lays down too much collagen, resulting in damage to blood vessels, skin, joints and some of the internal organs. About 1,500 people in the UK are affected by it.

Raynaud's phenomenon commonly accompanies scleroderma. This is a situation in which the blood vessels of the hands and feet go into spasm to produce painful, itching and cold extremities.

Sjögren's syndrome

Sjögren's syndrome is another auto-immune condition, in which the moisture-producing glands of the body are attacked. This produces dry eyes, dry mouth and joint pains. Other internal organs can be affected. There are about 500,000 people affected in the UK.

Septic arthritis

Septic arthritis occurs when there is a direct infection of a joint, most commonly the hip or the knee. It can affect people of any age, but is more common in the elderly and in young children, particularly under the age of five years. They can be quite unwell with it. The treatment is that of the underlying infection.

Lyme disease

Lyme disease is spread by a tick called *Borellia burgdorferi*. It produces a characteristic fever and a 'bull's-eye' type of rash on the upper arm, leg or trunk anywhere between 3 and 30 days after a tick bite. Arthritis and other problems can be associated with it. The treatment is a course of the appropriate antibiotic.

Gout

Hippocrates referred to gout as 'the disease of kings' because of its association with a rich diet. Later physicians called it *opprobium medicorum*, 'the reproach of physicians', because it was so difficult to treat. It is a crystal arthritis – crystals of uric acid form in a joint to produce inflammation and severe pain. It is commonest in the big toe joints, the wrists and the knees. Uric acid crystals can also form in the kidneys to produce loin pain.

Gout is commoner in males, in a ratio of 5:1. It is more likely in people who are overweight, who drink excessive alcohol, who consume a high protein diet or who are on certain drugs. However, there is a genetic predisposition, and by no means everyone who gets it is guilty of over-indulgence.

It is treated with anti-inflammatory agents or a drug called colchicine. In many people the drug allopurinol is used as a preventative treatment.

4

Rheumatism

Guillaume de Baillou (1538–1616), a French physician and Dean of the Faculty of Medicine at the University of Paris, was the first person to use the word 'rheumatism' and to describe arthritis, in a treatise published in 1578 and entitled *Liber de Rheumatismo et Pleuritide dorsali*. This was really the first book devoted to the subject.

'Rheumatism' was a non-specific term, just as it remains a non-specific term today. In general, however, it is used to describe those conditions affecting the soft tissues of the locomotor system.

Polymyalgia rheumatica

Polymyalgia rheumatica is an inflammatory condition affecting the muscles. The name *polymyalgia* means 'pain in many muscles'. Marked stiffness is also present. It occurs above the age of 50 and affects females more than males. It classically affects the muscles of the shoulder and pelvic girdles, so that certain movements, like brushing or washing one's hair or getting up out of a chair, become difficult and painful.

The onset can be sudden, in that it seems to come out of the blue one morning when one wakes with pain and stiffness in many muscles, but especially around the shoulders and the pelvis. The pattern continues with pains and stiffness that are worse in the mornings. Turning over in bed can be difficult and the person feels tired all the time, as if she has been overworking her muscles. It is common to feel down in the dumps and depressed. Some people lose weight.

This condition may seem similar to rheumatoid arthritis, but a physical examination by your doctor will usually differentiate the two. A blood test is vital to check the ESR. This will be very high, suggesting the presence of a lot of inflammation. The treatment is a course of corticosteroids. Most people notice an incredible improvement when they are first put on them, and the blood test usually mirrors this, in that the ESR will come tumbling back down. It is likely that the corticosteroids will need to be continued at a maintenance dosage for some months, and in some people for a year or two, or relapse can occur.

Treatment is important because it is possible for a quarter of all cases of polymyalgia rheumatica to merge into another very serious condition – temporal arteritis – which we shall now consider.

Temporal arteritis

Note that this is not a type of arthritis, but an inflammatory condition of arteries. These are the blood vessels that carry blood from the heart to all the parts of the body. Hence the word 'arteritis', indicating inflammation of an artery, rather than 'arthritis'. This condition classically affects the temporal arteries, the main arteries at the temples, although it can affect any of the arteries supplying the scalp and the head and neck. Most significantly, it can affect the arteries that supply the eyes, with the possibility of sudden loss of vision and possible blindness. It affects the same age group as polymyalgia rheumatica. It is rare under the age of 50.

The condition is also known as giant cell arteritis, because of the particular types of cells that are found on biopsy of the affected blood vessel.

The typical symptoms are of severe throbbing headache, usually one-sided, associated with scalp tenderness. There may also be facial pain, pain on moving the tongue and disturbance of vision. All of these are really emergency symptoms and merit an urgent medical opinion.

Treatment with corticosteroids can prevent blindness. The stark fact is that 30–50 per cent of people with this condition experience visual problems before diagnosis, so it is important to receive treatment before permanent blindness occurs.

Fibromyalgia syndrome

This complex condition can be confused with polymyalgia rheumatica, and it has provoked a great deal of controversy in medical circles. It is characterized by great pain anywhere from head to toe, often flitting in nature, muscle stiffness and fatigue. The pains can be continuous or there can be exquisitely painful spasms. It is commonest between the ages of 40 and 50 years, and more than 90 per cent of people with fibromyalgia are female. All the usual rheumatological tests tend to be normal.

At one time medical opinion was that it was a stress condition. This was because it often, although not always, seems to stem from some triggering illness or stress. Thankfully, times have changed and it is now recognized as a very real and at times debilitating condition.

People may experience a number of symptoms, including:

- muscle pain;
- stiffness;
- tender trigger points in muscles;
- muscle spasms;
- fatigue;
- poor concentration and muddled thinking;
- headaches; and
- emotional changes, such as anxiety and depression.

In addition, people often have symptoms from related conditions such as irritable bowel syndrome and irritable bladder syndrome. They may also be subject to allergies and various other nuisance symptoms.

The diagnosis is made on the basis of a history of bilateral pain, pain both above and below the pelvis, and pain along the spine, as well as the presence of 11 or more painful trigger points over various muscles. Incidentally, many of these trigger points overlap traditional acupuncture points. In practice, the diagnosis is more one of exclusion. In other words, it is made once the doctor has excluded the inflammatory arthropathies and conditions like polymyalgia rheumatica.

Treatment includes the use of pain-killers, antidepressants and, increasingly, a multi-disciplinary approach. The use of antidepressants can be helpful both to combat depression and also to raise the pain threshold.

Tendinitis

As discussed in Chapter 2, on the locomotor system, tendons are fibrous bands that attach muscles to bones. They can become inflamed and produce much pain, tenderness and limitation of movement. Corticosteroid injections or a treatment like acupuncture may help dramatically. There are several common sites of tendinitis.

Shoulder tendinitis

There are several tendons around the shoulder joint. These form the rotator cuff, a group of muscles that move the shoulder joint. Any of them can become inflamed. The commonest ones to be inflamed are the supraspinatus tendon at the front of the shoulder and the infraspinatus at the back of the shoulder.

Golfer's elbow and tennis elbow

These are two conditions that cause elbow pain. The medical name for golfer's elbow is medial epicondylitis, because it causes pain on the inside of the elbow. For tennis elbow the medical name is lateral epicondylitis, because there is inflammation of the point of insertion of the tendon into the epicondyle on the outside of the elbow. Neither really has much to do with the respective sports they are named after, but both cause pain when using the muscles that attach to the tendons. Golfer's elbow produces pain inside the elbow when the flexor muscles are used to bend the wrist and flex the fingers. Tennis elbow produces pain on the outside of the elbow when the wrist is extended and the muscles fingers are straightened. Pouring movements often cause pain.

Thumb tendinitis

This is the condition of de Quervain's tenosynovitis. It is an inflammation of the tendons that operate the thumb as they run through lubricated anatomical sheaths.

Patellar tendinitis

Patellar tendinitis causes pain below the kneecap. It can occur in youngsters between ten and 14 years, and also in athletes.

Achilles tendinitis

Achilles tendinitis causes pain in the back of the ankle at the point where the Achilles tendon joins the gastrocnemius (calf muscle) to the back of the calcaneus or heel bone. It is often caused by a sporting strain. If it occurs it needs rest and one should not try to work through it. The danger is of actually ending up with a tear or a rupture of the tendon.

Repetitive strain injury

Repetitive strain injury is the name for a group of conditions that may affect the muscles, tendons and joints of the spine, upper and lower limbs. As the name suggests it is the result of repeated movements that produce strain on the parts moved. It can occur as a result of sport or work, or from using any type of tool over and over again.

Treatment

Treatment involves understanding the mechanism of the pain, appropriate rest, possibly physiotherapy and stretching. Again, many people may respond to corticosteroid injections or acupuncture.

Bursitis

Bursitis is inflammation of one or more of the bursae around a joint. As mentioned in Chapter 2, the bursae are small synovial lined sacs around joints. There are about 160 of them in the body. When the synovial fluid inside a bursa becomes infected, or if the membranes become inflamed from too much movement having taken place or too much pressure on them, the bursa can become inflamed. The bursa often produces swelling of the part, and pain when pressure is put on it. This is the condition of bursitis. There are various places where this is common:

- Sub-acromial bursitis and deltoid bursitis, producing pain around the shoulder.
- Olecranon bursitis, producing pain around the point of the elbow.
- Trochanteric bursitis, producing pain around the outside of the hip.
- Popliteal bursitis – housemaid's knee or clergyman's knee – producing pain around the knee.

The recommended treatment can be summed up by the letters P–R–I–C–E–M, standing for protection, rest, ice, compression, elevation and medication. The medication usually consists of anti-inflammatory drugs and possibly corticosteroid injection into the bursa.

Nerve entrapment syndromes

There are various painful conditions that result from nerves becoming compressed or entrapped at various vulnerable points in the extremities or as they run through various anatomical tunnels.

Carpal tunnel syndrome

Carpal tunnel syndrome results from entrapment of the median nerve as it passes through the carpal tunnel in the wrist. It produces pain, pins and needles, and numbness in the thumb, index finger and middle fingers.

Cubital tunnel syndrome

Cubital tunnel syndrome results from inflammation of the ulnar nerve as it passes through a small tunnel behind the elbow. This is actually the nerve that you hit if you bump your 'funny bone'. This is a condition that is sometimes confused with golfer's elbow. Its common name is 'mobile phone elbow.' It is associated with pain, numbness and tingling down the inside of the arm to the ring and little finger.

Sciatica

Sciatica is an entrapment of the sciatic nerve (the main nerve of the leg) or of one or more of its nerve roots. It can be very debilitating and is often associated with low back pain. Pains radiate all the way down the leg, the exact distribution giving a useful indication of which nerve roots are affected. There is usually difficulty in lifting the leg.

Meralgia paraesthetica

Meralgia paraesthetica is a specific nerve entrapment of the lateral cutaneous nerve of the thigh. It causes pain, pins and needles and numbness of the outer surface of the thigh.

Treatment

The treatment of nerve entrapment syndromes usually involves rest, physiotherapy and medication. In prolonged cases accurate diagnosis is necessary, entailing detailed investigations. In the case of sciatica, for example, the cause could be a prolapsed intervertebral disc. Surgery may be necessary.

Chronic low back pain

Low back pain is a potential problem for everyone. One might think that the diagnosis would be simple, yet some people, despite intensive investigations, are left with intractable low back pain. Some probably have some degree of fibromyalgia. Others are simply diagnosed as having mechanical back pain, which is a way of saying that no one knows why they have it.

There is always something that the person can do with self-help to improve this problem.

Borderline rheumatics

In a similar way to chronic back pain, some people have all the features of some of the conditions I have mentioned, yet no firm diagnosis can be made. They may be given reassurance, but that does not always help. Some will go on to develop one of the arthritic conditions or finally be diagnosed with fibromyalgia. In the old days they were simply told that they had rheumatics. Again, there is much that self-help can do for pain and stiffness.

Osteoporosis

Osteoporosis is an extremely important condition to have correctly diagnosed. It is commonly known as 'thinning of the bones.' It is considered in this chapter because it is not an arthritic condition, but merits consideration on its own. In osteoporosis the bone mineral density (BMD) is reduced as a result of loss of calcium, so that the bone architecture is disrupted, the bones are less dense and fractures are more likely. It is commonest in post-menopausal women. It is certainly the commonest bone disorder in the elderly and affects at least 20 per cent of women by the age of 70 years.

Certain bones are more vulnerable than others. Indeed, a fracture is often the first time that it is diagnosed. The lower radius can fracture in a Colles' wrist fracture in women in their 50s; the scaphoid is also a common site of fracture. Both these types of fracture can occur when you fall and try to save yourself by stretching your hand in front of you to break the fall. Fracture of the hip can occur in the 60s, and fractures of the spinal vertebrae, known as 'crush fractures' can occur from 70 years and upwards. Crush fractures – rather like a toasted marshmallow being crushed – are extremely painful. They tend to result in a slow and progressive hunching forward to produce the characteristic 'dowager's hump'.

There are established criteria for diagnosing those at risk of osteoporosis, relating to the bone density as assessed with a DEXA scan, which can be arranged through one's GP. The aim is to prevent osteoporosis reaching a point where fractures are likely. We have very effective drugs such as alendronate, etidronate, risedronate, raloxifene and strontium ranelate. In addition, it is a good idea for all women over the age of 40 to take a daily calcium and vitamin D tablet.

5

The enigma of pain

Pain is an enigma. It is not an actual entity itself, but an experience that is unique to the individual. You cannot, after all, 'feel someone's pain'. And you cannot bring a pain back to mind when it has gone. You can recall that it was unpleasant, perhaps extremely unpleasant, yet you cannot reproduce it once it has gone. Now, that is an interesting point.

It is important to differentiate acute from chronic pain. Many people mistakenly think that acute and chronic are two poles of a spectrum of experience. This is not the case. They are two entirely different types of pain.

'Acute' pain is the expected physiological response to a stimulation that is immediately perceived as being noxious or unpleasant to the body. The simplest example is the immediate reflex withdrawal of your hand when you burn your fingers. If the burn is mild the pain will go in a relatively short period of time. This type of pain is seen to have a purpose, in that it alerts the body to a problem that it can readily relieve. It causes the person to take action to avoid further injury or damage.

'Chronic' pain, on the other hand, is the continual experience of an unpleasant sensation that is unlikely to disappear of its own accord. This is the typical background chronic pain of arthritis. Unlike acute pain, it should be clear that this type of pain has no useful function. It just grinds away at you and can, if you allow it, impair your quality of life. Clearly, coping with chronic pain can be difficult, since it is hard to ignore pain. Indeed, in some people the intensity can be such that pain seems to dominate their life. This is something that you must not allow to happen.

Pain theories

When I was a medical student we were taught that pain was the result of nerve stimulation and that it could be understood in the same manner that one could understand a circuit diagram.

Pain pathways

We start with the stimulation. All over and throughout the body you have tiny sensors called nociceptors. The word is derived from the Latin *nocere*, 'to injure'. We have known about them since 1906, when Sir Charles Scott Sherrington, professor of physiology at Oxford University and a Nobel laureate, first described them. These nociceptors basically react to all injurious or harmful stimuli.

The first effect of the stimulus is to create pressure on this nerve-end nociceptor. For example, temperature at the site may be increased and the tissues will release a whole range of chemicals into the tissue fluid that surrounds the nociceptor, which will start an impulse up the nerve.

We were taught that it was just a question of knowing about the circuits involved. In this example of an injury to the skin, impulses would pass along the nerves to reach the spinal cord. The nerve impulses would pass upwards along a pain pathway to the spinal cord, and then pass up into the brain, where they would reach a pain centre. This special pain centre would perceive the stimulus and the person would

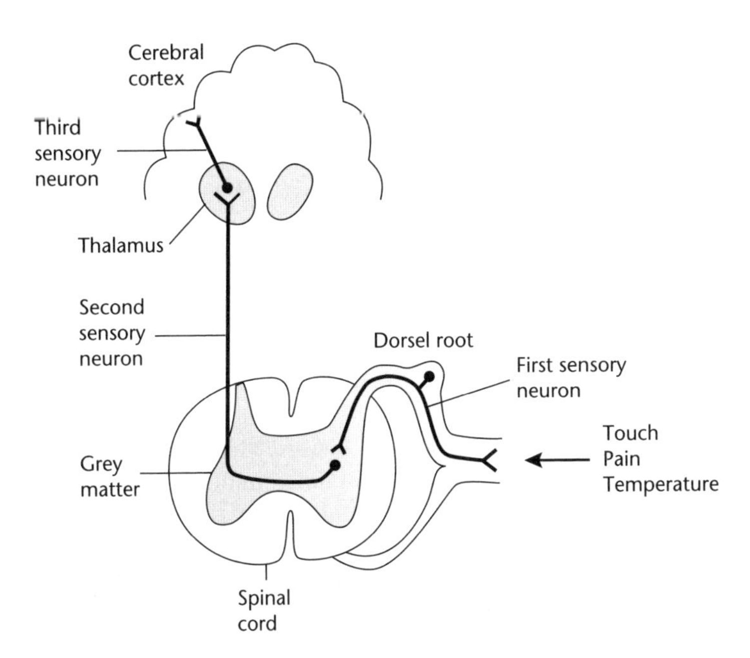

Figure 5.1 What happens when a painful stimulus is received

'feel the pain'. The site of this so-called pain centre was open to much debate over the decades, some suggesting that it was in the cerebral cortex (the 'thinking part' of the brain) and others suggesting that it was in the thalamus at the top of the brainstem. But all in all, although the exact site of the pain centre was unknown, it was taught that it was all rather like the circuitry for operating a doorbell, with the final experience of pain likened to the noise of the doorbell ringing.

Several of these pathways have been described and are well recognized. I will consider just one, which will give you a good idea of how a pain pathway works. This is the spinothalamic tract (see Figure 5.1, page 37).

Figure 5.1 illustrates what happens when a painful stimulus is received. The stimulus passes along nerves up to the spinal cord, which is shown in section at the bottom of the diagram. A neurone or nerve cell transmits this from the dorsal horn of the spinal cord and crosses over to the opposite side of the cord, where it joins with another neurone, which transmits the impulse up the cord to the thalamus at the base of the brain. Another neurone takes the impulse *upwards to higher centres*, where the pain is perceived.

The spinothalamic tract carries nerve fibres that are responsible for transmitting information about pain, fine touch and temperature. So, depending upon which type of fibres within a nerve are stimulated, the person may feel pain, fine touch or the sensation of heat or cold.

If the stimulus was very light, the fine touch fibres would be selectively stimulated, so that a tickle would be felt. If the stimulus was slightly stronger, some pain fibres and some fine touch fibres would be stimulated, so that an itch would be perceived. If the temperature fibres were also stimulated, a sensation of heat (or cold) would be felt. And if the stimulus was very strong, pain would be felt, possibly also being perceived as burning pain or itching pain.

All of this fits the experience of acute pain, because the stimulus produces a sensation, the brain causes a behaviour to remove the part from the source of the pain, and ultimately the pain should subside.

So far so good, but chronic pain seemed much more complex to understand. And it still is. It seems that different nerve fibres get stimulated and that somehow they retain a memory of that stimulation. It is almost as if the pain memory gets stuck and it replays itself, stimulated again and again. Yet it is more complex than even that. It became clear that chronic pain, from conditions like arthritis, cannot be explained just on the basis of these nerve pathways. There seemed to be a chemical component as the result of inflammation.

Tissue damage and inflammation

Inflammation is one of the main mechanisms of pain in arthritis and rheumatism. As mentioned above, tissue damage causes the release of the body's own chemicals into the tissue fluid that surrounds and bathes the nociceptors. Neighbouring cells, called mast cells, release other pain-producing and inflammation-inducing chemicals into the area. There are many types of these chemicals that have been identified, including bradykinin, histamine, prostaglandins, leukotrienes, various peptides and proteolytic enzymes. All can induce pain and stimulate the nociceptors and nerve endings. They are discussed further in Chapter 11, which considers anti-inflammatory oils and nutrition.

Once inflammation gets started, it produces dilatation of the blood vessels to produce redness and leaking from the vessels to cause tissue fluid accumulation and swelling around the area.

The gate control theory of pain

In 1965 a psychologist, Dr Ronald Melzack, and a physician and neuroscientist, Dr Patrick Wall (both of whom became professors), published their quite revolutionary gate theory of pain. This theory postulated a series of pain pathways and the means by which chronic pain could be perceived and modified. Melzack and Wall suggested that a series of 'gates' in the spinal cord could be opened (to perceive pain) or closed (to block it). These gates could be blocked by descending messages from the brain. Effectively this explained the way that psychological functions of the brain could have a bearing on the experience of pain. Thus, anxiety, depression and other negative emotions can open the gates to allow pain to be perceived, or even worsen it. So too can the physical side of life, such as inactivity, getting too tired or overdoing it. On the other hand, factors such as auto-suggestion (see page 73), talking therapies and various types of distraction may close the gates to diminish pain.

This was immensely helpful in understanding painful conditions and opened up a whole new area of research, which has seen the development of a speciality in pain management and the flourishing of pain clinics.

Neurotransmitters and endorphins

In 1921, Dr Otto Loewi, an Austrian scientist, discovered a chemical in tissue that we now call acetylcholine, which was released into the blood stream and which could affect nerve tissue. This was the first of the chemicals to be discovered that we now call neurotransmitters. There are several ways of classifying neurotransmitters, but for our purposes it is sufficient to know that there are amino acids, peptides and monoamines. They tend to be either excitatory or inhibitory in action. Many are involved in the mechanism of pain production.

Serotonin, or 5-hydroxytryptamine (5-HT), is one of the neurotransmitters. It is built from the amino acid tryptamine, and has been called the 'happiness neurotransmitter'. When levels are low the person can feel depressed, hence the use of a class of antidepressant drugs called the selective serotonin reuptake inhibitors (SSRIs), which work by keeping the level of serotonin constant.

In the 1970s a group of naturally occurring chemicals called endorphins were independently discovered by Roger Guillemin and Andrew W. Schally, who were awarded the 1977 Nobel Prize for their work. These are a type of protein molecule that have a similar action to opiates. They can therefore lift the spirits and seem to alleviate the experience of pain. Various foods such as chocolate and chillies, exercise, many types of physical therapy and acupuncture have all been shown to cause endorphin release.

Another interesting neurotransmitter is a protein called substance P. This was originally discovered in 1931, but recently it has been found to have a significant role in conditions like fibromyalgia, chronic back pain, and arthritis and rheumatism. It seems to be involved in inflammation and pain perception, and it is also involved in the control of moods and anxiety levels. Capsaicin, derived from chillies, is known to reduce tissue levels of substance P when it is applied regularly as an ointment.

Phantom limb pain

Phantom limb pain has always been a difficult phenomenon to explain. People who have lost limbs or who have been born without limbs often experience pain in the missing limb. The pain they experience is very real, but very difficult to deal with. At one time it was assumed that it was a psychologically induced pain, since there were no tissues to produce the pain. Yet this strange phenomenon actually points to a different explanation, which is that the brain is not just a sensor and analyser of incoming information from the extremities, but it contains all the apparatus to perceive the whole body even if someone is born without a part of it.

This is very logical, if you think of the way that we develop from a few cells into a ball of cells, gradually folding parts in here and there, in a set pattern until a body shape is developed, with all tissues in the right place and all organs formed and set to work according to their predetermined function. Essentially, it is part of the hard-wiring of the brain.

This analysis was to lead on to the most exciting theory of pain, in terms of its potential to ultimately alleviate pain.

The human pain matrix

With the development of various types of scanners it has become possible to research pain in a way that was not possible 20 years ago. Two types of scan have helped – functional magnetic resonance imaging (fMRI) and positive emission tomography (PET). These scans now enable scientists to see what is happening to various parts of the brain while people are performing different tasks or thinking different thoughts. This has dramatically improved our understanding of painful conditions.

We now understand that the perception of pain is not just a matter of nerve circuitry, but involves neurotransmitter release, the opening and closing of neural gates, the localization of pain in the brain, and the influence of thought patterns, emotions and even life situations. This is phenomenally important in terms of helping a person to influence the pain he or she feels.

The concept of the human pain matrix is now well established. It is accepted that the brain itself holds information about how the body should look, how it should operate, and how it analyses information from the body. The contribution of the mind, the thought processes and the emotions is seen to be of fundamental importance within this matrix.

This pain matrix has two components, which operate in parallel. The innermost, called the medial pain system, processes the emotional side of pain. This includes fear, anxiety and stress. The outermost, or the lateral pain system, seems to be responsible for processing the physical sensations, such as the intensity of the pain, its localization in the body, and its duration.

Experiments with PET scans have shown that different parts of the pain matrix light up[6] when people are experiencing a flare-up of genuine pain as opposed to artificially induced pain using heat. Artificial pain will predominantly affect the lateral pain system, whereas a flare-up of arthritic knee pain will light up the medial system as well as the lateral system. The implication is that the emotional side is operant because the person's mind will recall the pain, will associate memories with it and will process it as the person worries if it is going to deteriorate or follow the recognized pattern.

The importance of all this is that it implies that there may be several different ways of attacking chronic pain. It is no longer simply a matter of trying to block a nerve pathway, or of affecting a level of a chemical in the body, but of adopting a multiple or multi-dimensional approach. And once again that means that people can do so much, because it is their brain, their body, their lifestyle and their life that is being affected. You can see from this why the life cycle approach (see Chapter 1) can be very relevant.

Pain in arthritis and rheumatism

It is not always clear why people experience pain in many of these conditions. For example, although osteoarthritis affects the integrity and structure of the cartilage, cartilage has no nerve fibres in it. There are several mechanisms that can be considered, including irritation from debris from joint damage, crystal formation in joints, immunological reactions, chemical mediators of inflammation like histamine, increased pressure within joints, and pressure upon the bones themselves. Yet in addition to these possible causes, it is important also to consider the theories of pain and the human pain matrix in terms of how that pain is perceived.

In rheumatoid arthritis and the inflammatory arthropathies, the mechanism seems to relate very much to inflammation. All the methods that can be used to reduce inflammation (including drug treatment, cooling, various supplements and nutritional changes) therefore have a large part to play.

Fibromyalgia is a condition that has baffled doctors for decades. The pain does not relate to inflammatory markers, as do the inflammatory arthropathies, yet there is no doubt that pain is a dominant feature. The factors I mentioned above are important, but the state of the ligaments, the muscles and the muscle fibres that make up the muscle bulk seem to be the source of the pain. Micro-injuries to muscle fibres, tension within the muscles and the changes that come about through stiffness are all important. Indeed, when a muscle becomes stiff it starts to send off a pain signal of its own. You can imagine that when a muscle contracts and is held in a state of contraction, it will develop cramp. And much of the pain of fibromyalgia feels at times like an exaggerated cramp. This is considered in Chapter 6, on stiffness.

Remember, you can't study fish out of water

Modern science is reductionist. We take things apart and look at the parts, and we look at how those parts are made up. Medicine as one of the natural sciences is also reductionist, in that it is practised according to systems of the body. Hence you have dermatologists specializing in skin disorders and rheumatologists mainly specializing in disorders of the locomotor system. And in our discussion of pain we have looked at it in terms of neuro-circuits and neurotransmitters. Yet as we have also seen, the perception of pain is very complex, and the mind cannot be taken out of the equation. It is your mind, conscious or unconscious, that has a part to play in opening or closing the gates in the spinal cord. Likewise, when parts of the human pain matrix are stimulated, they will trigger associations from memory, the emotions and the higher thinking brain, which will have a great part to play in the process of pain perception.

Yet it is in fact even more complex than that. Whereas at one time biologists were happy to examine living creatures anatomically and physiologically, they later came to realize that you cannot know all about them without studying their environment. Hippocrates, the father of medicine, wrote a treatise in the 5th century BC entitled *Airs, Waters and Places*, in which he taught that a physician must study the air that men breathe, the waters they drink and the place that they live their lives. This was profound, and its wisdom is very relevant today. In order to understand how a condition affects someone, it is important to know how it affects him or her in the five spheres of the life cycle.

Vicious circle of pain

Often pain is at the root of a problem as well as being the result. Again, considering the five spheres, you can see that a continuous or recurrent pain can make you anxious or depressed. When you feel anxious or depressed it alters your thought processes, which generally become negative, fearful or full of dread. This in turn can make you less active, isolated and reclusive. This can have a significant impact on your life, your work and your relationships. And because of this you can dwell on it, which directly affects your pain matrix so that the pain is intensified, the control gates stay open and you are back at square one. What happens is a tendency to spiral downwards, and the condition takes more and more control of your life.

Pain and the life cycle

It is worth getting out your exercise book again and, under a fresh heading of 'Pain', looking at the symptom of pain and going through the five spheres to see how pain itself is affecting your life. Is it different from the first life cycle drawing you made?

The important point of the exercise is to show that pain is not just a thing that you can only deal with by taking a tablet. Look at all those arrows. Essentially the life cycle is showing you that there are several potential interventions at all these levels to help you deal with it.

Pain diary

It is certainly worth keeping a record of your pain – a pain diary. You can either record it in a separate section of your exercise book or actually get a diary and monitor your pain levels each day. I suggest that you score pain on a range from 0 to 10, where 0 is no pain and 10 is the worst pain imaginable (the pain that you imagine you would experience from being boiled in oil, perhaps).

At the top of each page, put headings as shown in Table 5.1 and mark out a series of columns running through each day. I find this is a useful way of looking at what you are doing and it helps to reinforce the way of examining things in terms of the life cycle.

There are several ways that you can record your pain diary. You can leave it all to the end of the day and record a summary, but this is in my view the least helpful. I suggest that a more useful way is to make a record each time you are aware of a marked level of pain. Or, if you prefer, just select three times of the day and record it.

In the *Date* column, write date and the time of each recording. Under *Body*, focus on the pain and write down its level. Under *Emotions*, record how the pain made you feel (e.g. sad, angry, anxious). Under

Table 5.1 Headings for each page of a pain diary

Date	*Body*	*Emotions*	*Mind*	*Behaviour*	*Questions*

Mind write down what you thought, (e.g. 'Oh dear!', 'Oh no!', 'This is terrible!'). Under *Behaviour*, write down what you were doing at the time (e.g. exercising, gardening, working on the computer) and what you did about it (e.g. nothing, took a pain-killer, made tea, stretched). You can score your pain level after you took that action.

Leave the *Questions* column blank for now, because this is something that you can come back to. Indeed, I shall return to this when we come to Chapter 8, on emotions and mind matters.

After a week or so you may see if a pattern has developed. You will see if certain things worsen or provoke your pain. And you may see what behaviour or action could improve it.

Drugs

Now for many people drugs will be an important part of keeping their condition under control. I do not decry them, for as a conventionally trained doctor I have used them all in my practice.

There are basically four types of drugs used to control pain.

1 Analgesics or pain-killers. These include drugs such as aspirin, paracetamol, codeine, dihydrocodeine, tramadol and morphine. They vary immensely in strength. Common side effects are constipation, drowsiness, nausea and mood changes.
2 Anti-inflammatory drugs. These include the non-steroidal anti-inflammatory drugs (NSAIDs), such as ibuprofen, indomethacin and diclofenac. There are also stronger drugs like corticosteroids. Common side effects include gastric upsets, bleeding from the stomach or gut, and possibly worsening of asthma.
3 Antidepressants. The main ones used are amitriptyline and dothiepin. As pain controllers they are often used in a sub-antidepressant dose, since they are being used to alter the threshold of pain. Common side effects are palpitations, dry mouth, blurred vision, cramps, constipation and possibly retention of urine in men.
4 Anticonvulsants. These include carbamazepine and gabapentin. These drugs are really only used in intractable pain and may be prescribed in a pain clinic setting.

And of course there are also DMARDs, the disease-modifying anti-rheumatic drugs which I mentioned in Chapter 3. They are of inestimable value in rheumatoid arthritis and related types of arthritis.

When do you take a pain-killer?

This is a question I think that you ought to try focusing on, because many people end up taking far too many pain-killers. Indeed, it is well known that if you use pain-killers too often, you alter the threshold of pain and the level at which they work. I think that you should aim to take as few pain-killers as you can. That is not to say that you should stop them, but you ought to try working out a level of pain at which you should take one. Begin by working out what level of pain you feel that you can cope with, which may be about 3 on your scoring scale of 0 to 10. Work out what level is definitely unacceptable, probably 6 and above. But if you look at your pain diary you should start to see a pattern. And you will be able to rationalize when you take a pain-killer.

Other actions that may help

Rather than taking a pain-killer, you might consider the following:

- Do something interesting to distract yourself.
- If practicable, take a hot shower.
- Try a little stretching.
- If a part is feeling hot and painful, try cooling it with a cool pack and just rest for a while.
- Try a little massage or apply a rubefacient ointment.

TENS machines

Transcutaneous electrical nerve stimulation (TENS) machines are portable machines that deliver small electrical impulses to the body from a battery pack, via wires, to electrodes strapped over a painful part. They can be useful but should be used only after a proper diagnosis and proper instructions as to their use. They should not be used if you are pregnant (unless advised by your doctor), have a pacemaker, or have epilepsy or certain heart conditions. In short, it is best to seek a face-to-face medical opinion as to whether they would be helpful or not.

Your imagination is a powerful pain-killer

Now it is time to start using your imagination to see if you can control some of your pain.

Back in 2002 I attended an interesting and thought-provoking art exhibition at St Thomas' Hospital in London. The theme was chronic pain. It was really a very clever idea, because of the difficulty people have in describing their pain. As I have mentioned before, pain is a bit of an enigma.

The photographs in the exhibition were portrayals of people's perceptions of their pain. One image was of a concrete strait-jacket, illustrating one person's experience and perception of pain. To this person the pain was a solid thing, a constricting and an isolating thing. And there is that isolation concept again. The concrete weighs you down. Other photographs showed red-hot wires glowing in the dark, animal scratches on stone, and gloves full of crawling ants. You can imagine the types of pain those people were experiencing. It is really the quality of the pain that they are describing.

The imagery is fascinating, because this is something that is worth trying out right now. Try to imagine what your pain looks like in a symbolic manner. It is the quality of the pain that I want you to think about.

If you can do that, you can modify it. For example, if you have a pain in your back like a tight band, or a taut rope, close your eyes and visualize that rope with a great big tight knot in it. Focus hard and mentally try to loosen the knot. Or you may feel a burning pain, which you may imagine as a smouldering cord. Picture it in your mind as it is soaked in water, extinguishing the fire. Or if you have imagined a cold pain as an icicle, imagine it being warmed up, gradually melting away.

It is worth letting your creativity conjure up the image of the symptom that you have. Sit or lie down and make yourself as comfortable as you can, somewhere that you will not be disturbed. Let your mind throw up images that seem right, and when you have the image that corresponds best with the pain, use your mind to reverse the effect. As you do this so you tell yourself that you are reducing it, lessening the discomfort until it goes.

Your mind is very powerful and it is worth making it work for you. It is all part of taking control, as I implied at the outset. Try doing this every day for a week. You may be very surprised at the results. And that is a start. We shall return to this later when we look at self-hypnosis and relaxation techniques in Chapter 12, on complementary medicine.

Key points

- Understanding how pain affects you can help to alleviate it.
- Use the life cycle to see what changes in the five spheres could help you reduce your pain level.
- Start a pain diary.
- Rationalize your use of pain-killers – be able to say at what level you need a pain-killer.
- Start to use your imagination as a pain reliever.
- Consider other things that may lessen your discomfort.

6

Stiffness

Stiffness is one of the main problems of many rheumatic conditions. This can be stiffness of the joints themselves or stiffness of the surrounding soft tissues, or a combination of both. Stiffness can have several different mechanisms and it can be acute, chronic or acute on top of chronic.

Morning stiffness

Morning stiffness is very common in osteoarthritis, rheumatoid arthritis and some of the inflammatory arthropathies. In osteoarthritis it occurs first thing in the morning but quickly goes as one starts to move about. It rarely lasts for 30 minutes. In rheumatoid arthritis, it can be a real problem and may last longer than 45 minutes. When stiffness is a real problem in the mornings it is important to see your doctor to determine whether rheumatoid arthritis or one of the inflammatory arthropathies is causing the problem.

Painful stiffness

When stiffness is continuous and associated with pain, it is important to know what sort of problem you are dealing with. This is because joints are precious and you do not want to try to work an acutely inflamed joint by stoically working through the pain. That can cause further damage to the joint. Joint protection must always be one of your aims in self-help. I shall go into this in greater depth in Chapter 9, on lifestyle. Here I want to go through the nature of stiffness.

When the pain is just in the muscles, you do not have to be so wary, although a word of caution with the back. If after an acute strain a back pain is slow to resolve, and there is limitation of function or associated sciatic pain with pain on lifting the legs, there may be an underlying problem such as a prolapsed disc. A medical opinion would be indicated.

In general, you have to be sensible. And this is why it is important to have a diagnosis to start with and to understand the way that a condition can affect you. Essentially, joints are precious, while muscles do not need quite so much pampering.

I divide stiffness into four types:

1 Acute stiffness of a joint due to inflammation. This is typical of rheumatoid arthritis. The joint can become swollen and tender and hot to the touch, with reduction of movement.
2 Acute stiffness after an injury. This is common in muscles, especially after strenuous exertion or even mild exertion of muscles that have not been used for some time. This can occur with a back strain. It can also occur with joints, and it indicates that rest is needed to prevent further damage.
3 Protective locking of muscles. Another type of stiffness can occur when muscles contract and stay in a 'locked' state of contraction. This can occur around a joint or in the back in order to splint the part or hold it in position to prevent further damage. When this happens for long enough it will produce cramp and cause its own pain. This can occur acutely, or happen repeatedly.
4 Progressive stiffening with loss of function of the part. This can happen when joints are continually damaged, or you try to work through the pain. Here the pain is warning you to rest the joint. It also occurs when tendons and ligaments have been inflamed or injured and they undergo healing. The healing results in collagen being laid down, often in a more haphazard pattern than the normal anatomy, so that it heals with less elasticity. The part can become shortened, pulling a joint out of shape to restrict movement and produce alteration in its structure and possibly cause some deformity.

Muscle stiffness

First of all let us look at the structure of a skeletal muscle in more detail than we did in Chapter 2. All skeletal muscles have the same basic structure, whether it is a big muscle like the calf muscle or a thin, fine muscle like any of the muscles of the hand. The whole muscle is covered in a connective tissue membrane called the endomysium or fascia. This endomysium protects the muscle from rubbing against other muscles and other anatomical structures. It extends beyond the muscle to form the fibrous tissue of a tendon, which anchors it to bone. Inside the endomysium the muscle is composed of bundles called fasciculi. Each bundle runs the length of the muscle and contains anything between ten and 100 muscle fibres. A muscle fibre is in fact a muscle cell. Each bundle is separated from another by more connective tissue called the

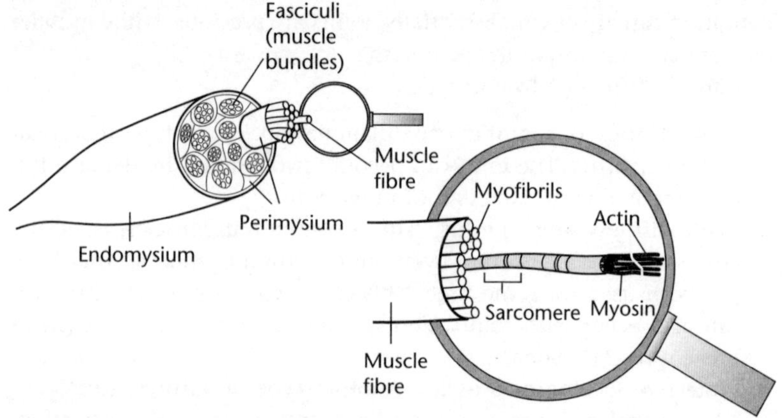

Figure 6.1 Structure of a muscle

perimysium. The number of bundles is dependent upon the type of muscle, so that the calf muscle has many and the finger muscles have few (Figure 6.1).

Each muscle fibre is like a long bag packed with smaller filament-like structures called myofibrils. It also contains a gel-like fluid called the sarcoplasm. It contains fats and glycogen and tiny structures called mitochondria, which collectively work as the powerhouse of the cell.

The sliding filament theory

Now, a little bit about how a muscle contracts. Within each myofibril there are even smaller, finer filaments called actin and mysosin micro-filaments. These are capable of sliding in and out during a muscle contraction. Each myofibril is composed of a whole chain of units called sarcomeres. A sarcomere is the smallest unit of a muscle that can contract. When it does so the actin and myosin slide over one another, as in Figure 6.2. This is the sliding filament theory, which explains how a muscle contracts and relaxes.

Thixotropy and stiffness

Thixotropy is the property that some gels or fluids have to become less viscous – less thick – when they are agitated or subjected to a shearing force. When the force is removed they can return to their original viscosity. Think of toothpaste in a tube: it is a gel inside the tube, but when you compress the sides of the tube, the toothpaste turns into a semi-fluid and oozes out of the tube, then resets on the toothbrush.

In a similar manner (although it is not quite thixotropic), tomato ketchup becomes a semi-solid when the bottle has been opened. A

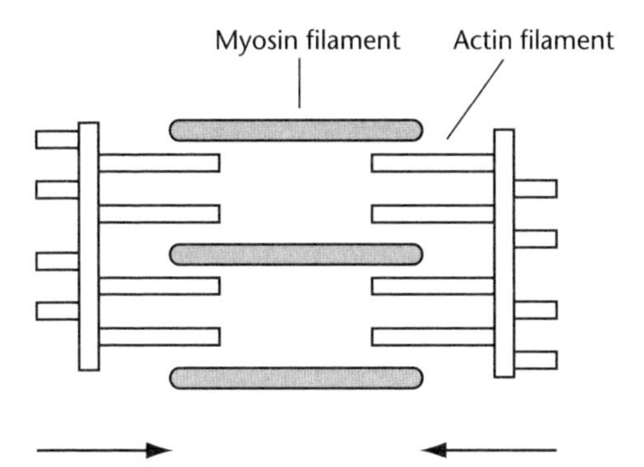

Figure 6.2 Actin and myosin microfilaments, which slide over each other as the muscle contracts or relaxes

half-full bottle can be an irritation because it simply will not pour. But if you tap the bottom of the bottle several times the ketchup will suddenly change from a semi-solid into a semi-liquid and a great dollop will come out.

Yet another example is quicksand. If you ever happen to find yourself in it (heaven forbid), you have to limit movement, because thrashing about makes this thixotropic substance become more fluid.

So what has all this to do with muscles? Well, the sacoplasma, the fluid in the myofibrils, is thixotropic. It can be semi-liquid or it can become quite viscous or gel-like. You can think of a muscle's structure as being like a bundle of long thin balloons filled with a substance like ketchup. When they are active, the fluid becomes semi-fluid and it moves well and produces a flexible muscle. When they are inactive and not used, the fluid becomes like the semi-solid ketchup that you see in an opened ketchup bottle. It is stiff and won't move well. But again, if you move it about, agitate it, it will become fluid again and flexible.

This seems to be one of the mechanisms of muscles stiffness. And so, please note, inactivity is the muscle's enemy. It makes the muscle go stiff.

Muscle locking

Sometimes muscles seem to lock and a part of the body just will not relax. This probably occurs because of bonding taking place between the sliding filaments – the actin and the myosin. It happens when contraction has occurred, possibly after an intense muscular contraction or a muscle spasm.

Imagine when you interlock your fingers (Figure 6.3 overleaf). The fingers slide between each other nice and easily. Slide them right up

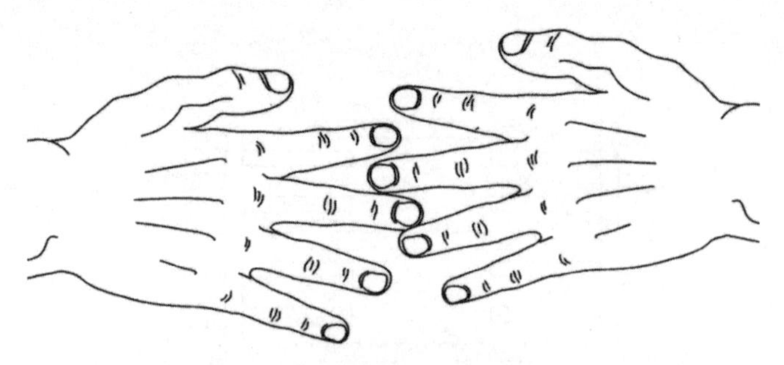

Figure 6.3 The way that our fingers can interlock is similar to the way that actin and myosin microfilaments slide over each other

together, to the finger webs. Now if you slightly flex the fingers and squeeze them together you find that they have 'locked'. The actin and mysosin are like opposing fingers. When they are apart but touching, that is like muscle relaxation. When they are interlaced, that is like muscle contraction. When they are 'locked', it is like locked muscle. This is analogous to the bonding that can form between the actin and myosin.

And this seems to be what happens when a muscle seizes up or locks. It will not let go until something allows it to release. Yet a locked muscle is not just an inert state. It uses up energy even doing nothing and it will eventually produce a cramp-like sensation and send out a pain signal.

Massage, gentle stretching, acupuncture and acupressure, and various manipulative therapies can all help to break down the stiffness and allow the muscles to relax.

Trigger points

All muscles have potential trigger points, little areas within the muscles that can become very tender. I mentioned some of them in Chapter 4, in the section on fibromyalgia. We are not precisely sure why these triggers develop, but they do seem to fit in with the picture of them being little locked segments of the muscle. Generally, when a trigger point becomes active, the whole muscle will contract down and pain will radiate along its length and to parts beyond it. This can produce what is called myofascial pain. If the trigger points are treated with some form of physical treatment, like massage, acupuncture or acupressure, the muscle will relax and the pain should decrease. Sometimes it can happen very dramatically, but sometimes several treatments are necessary.

These myofascial pains can sometimes cause a great deal of diagnostic confusion, in that, for example, sinusitis can be diagnosed when a trigger point in the jaw muscles is causing a pain that radiates over the facial sinuses. Similarly, migraine may be diagnosed when there are active trigger points in the temporalis muscle to produce pain that radiates up over the head. And trigger points in the gluteus muscles in the buttock may produce a pain that radiates down the leg, to produce a pseudo-sciatica.

Yet another important feature of these active trigger points is that, because the muscle is contracting, it will often alter the posture. Thus, triggers in the long paraspinal muscles may cause the spine to twist and lean in one direction. And gradually, if the problem is unrelieved, the posture changes and it can become very difficult to rectify.

Joint stiffness

Synovial fluid is also thixotropic. Now you can see how joints can become stiff if the synovial fluid becomes more viscous. This generally tends to occur with immobility, and so it is normal to be slightly stiff in the mornings.

In arthritis, the synovial fluid may be affected, increasing the thixotropic effect. And as the tendency to become less active sets in, the stiffening may increase.

Chronic stiffness

The connective tissue of the joints, ligaments and tendons and the perimysium of the muscles are all thixotropic, so all these structures are subject to the things discussed above. But on top of all this is the effect of healing to produce scar tissue. Scar tissue is always less elastic than the pre-injury or pre-damaged connective tissue. It will have the tendency to shorten and contract structures and hold them in a stiffer position. When there is much scar tissue the amount of elasticity that can be recovered is limited. But it is never too late to try to keep as supple as your body will permit, and in most cases this is more than you are allowing it to be at present.

Treatments

Heat and cold

Both heat and cold are useful for easing stiffness. Always be sure that you are applying it safely and be careful about applying either heat or cold directly to the skin. The skin can burn and can be easily damaged. Use a towel between a heat pack or a cold pack.

Heat from a wheat pack applied like this directly to the part will encourage dilatation of the blood vessels and improve the circulation. A cold pack will diminish inflammation and is useful if the part feels stiff and swollen. I generally advise five minutes of either at a time. Alternating from hot to cold to hot to cold to hot, five minutes each, is usually quite effective if stiffness is creating a real problem.

A sauna is an excellent type of treatment for stiffness. The dry heat of the sauna usually loosens up stiff muscles and joints. But you should always check with your doctor first if you have high blood pressure or a heart problem. Turkish baths supply moist heat and also seem to be beneficial to many people with rheumatism and arthritis. A sauna or Turkish bath once a week may help considerably if you can fit it into your schedule.

Self-massage

From what I have said about the mechanisms of stiffness, it is perhaps no surprise that I advocate self massage. I think that if you can get the muscles moving, you are liable to alter the thixotropic effect of both your muscles and joints. There are two things that I think are worth doing to help reduce stiffness each day.

Firstly, I recommend gentle patting or slapping of your body, starting at the feet and working up the legs, all over the trunk and up to the neck. Alternatively, do your arms from the hand up to the shoulder. It is most effective without clothes on before you have a bath or a shower in the morning. The whole thing takes just a minute or two, no more.

Secondly, I recommend dry brushing of the muscles. To do this, get a soft natural-fibre, long-handled brush or a long loofah. Brush gently all the muscles from the feet upwards, going over all the muscles with just a gentle stroking motion. Muscles seem to like this, and you are stimulating the circulation to the skin and also the lymphatic vessels beneath the skin. Spend ten minutes in the morning and then have a nice warm shower to clean off any dry skin.

Please note that you do it upwards in all cases, since you are doing it in the direction of the veins and the lymphatic system to encourage their flow. That way you will not work against them to risk damage to the valves in varicose veins.

Key points

- Understand the mechanisms of stiffness.
- Use heat and cold.
- Avoid inactivity.
- Practise self massage every morning.

7

Tiredness

Tiredness is an extremely common symptom in arthritis and many rheumatic conditions. It can have many causes and it is worth trying to pin down why you are tired, rather than just accepting it as something that you have to live with.

Possible causes of tiredness

Tiredness may be part of the condition

In some of the inflammatory conditions, such as rheumatoid arthritis, polymyalgia rheumatica and temporal arteritis, there is a lot happening chemically within the body. The inflammatory process throws a strain on the system, and tiredness results. When the inflammation is reduced, probably through anti-inflammatory treatment with NSAIDs, corticosteroids or one or other of the DMARDs, the energy levels should improve.

Tiredness may be due to anaemia

In rheumatoid arthritis it is not uncommon to develop anaemia. Anaemia means that there is a decrease in the number of red blood cells in the blood, that there is less haemoglobin in each red blood cell, or that there is abnormal haemoglobin. Haemoglobin is the oxygen-carrying protein in the red blood cells.

Iron deficiency is one of the commonest types of anaemia. It can result if not enough iron is taken in the diet, perhaps because of lack of appetite, but it also occurs if there is blood loss from the body. This can occur in some people when they take aspirin or any of the NSAIDs, such as ibuprofen or diclofenac. Always report excessive tiredness to your doctor, since a blood test can pin down the reason.

Lack of vitamin B12 is another cause of anaemia, and this too can be detected by blood testing.

Tiredness could be due to another condition

One cannot assume that all one's symptoms are due to the one that has been diagnosed. People do develop other conditions, such as hypothyroidism (underactivity of the thyroid gland), diabetes mellitus (when there may be excessive thirst and probably increased frequency of passage of urine) and problems such as inflammatory bowel disorders.

Tiredness could be due to the increased effort of it all

It is harder to do things when your muscles are painful and stiff, and when your joints are less mobile and stiff, as outlined in Chapter 7. If the stiffness is a result of the synovial fluid in your joints or the fluid in your muscle cells being more viscous, then the joints or muscles become harder to move. It requires more energy to do relatively simple tasks. Indeed, the more advanced the process is, the more energy you are expending in the simplest of actions in comparison to someone whose joints are fluid and whose muscles are sleek and efficient. Think of a bicycle that has been left in the garage over the winter. You wheel it out and try to cycle it, only to find the chain is dry, the gears are a bit rusted and the oil in the delicate parts is either dried up or very thick. If you try riding it you will expend much more energy than you would if you gave it a bit of maintenance and lubricated it.

Tiredness could be the interaction of pain and stiffness

Pain in itself can wear you down. It can effectively keep your mind on it, because it won't go away and you experience little relief. As we saw in the Chapter 5, on the enigma of pain, the pain matrix is very complex. It does not just transmit pain, but has all sorts of associations with past experience, old memories and with one's bank of emotions. If you can't switch off, you get exhausted.

Tiredness could be a consequence of immobility

It is a fact that the less mobile you are, the more it induces a tendency to become tired. The less you use muscles the less work they have to do, and they reduce in bulk. Incredibly, if you spend a whole day in bed, you will reduce muscle protein by eight grams. Over time the muscle tissue gets less and the fibrous tissue becomes a greater proportion of the muscle bulk. It is less flexible and less efficient and it tires more easily.

Joints become stiffer with less use, as I mentioned in Chapter 6. But the cardiovascular system will also be affected in a similar way, because the heart is a muscle and needs to be used. It will not wither away, but if you are inactive the heart becomes less adept at maintaining its output when you expect it to cope with an increased output, and the result will be quicker tiring.

It could be that you overdo it when you feel well

This is so common. I call it the dash-and-crash phenomenon. Because arthritis and rheumatism can vary, people often find that they have good days and bad days. When they have a good day they dash about trying to fit all sorts of things in. Very often these episodes of over-activity are followed by a pay-back. Energy levels plummet and the over-active period is followed by an episode when there is no energy left to do anything. Effectively, people crash out. Rather than being able to do your normal activities, it seems that you have to rest and be inactive. And at the same time you can get an aggravation of other symptoms, such as pain and stiffness.

The enforced rest sees a gradual return of energy, but it may seem to take longer each time, so that the rest periods have to get longer. As a result, you feel frustrated, and when your energy levels are reasonable again, on one of the good days, you just dash at it again. Hence one goes through cycles of dash and crash. This is a behaviour pattern that should be addressed and broken. But the first thing you have to do is recognize it!

Tiredness could be due to lack of sleep

As with any human parameter, it is hard to lay down numbers about ideal durations of sleep. Some people may sleep efficiently for six hours with no complaint, others need a full eight or nine hours of unbroken sleep. Insomnia is a highly subjective complaint. A reasonable working definition of insomnia is that it is 'a complaint of difficulty in initiating or maintaining satisfying sleep'.

Work in sleep laboratories over the last four decades has advanced our knowledge of the physiology of sleep. During a normal sleep time we seem to go through several cycles of sleep, composed of four stages of non-rapid eye movement (non-REM) and rapid eye movement (REM) sleep, in an ebb-and-flow manner (Figure 7.1 overleaf).

Non-REM sleep is divided into four progressively deeper stages: stage 1, or light sleep; stage 2, or middle sleep; and stages 3 and 4, deep or delta-wave sleep. REM sleep, when dreaming occurs, follows non-REM sleep and occurs in four or five episodes during a sleep time of about eight or nine hours. Generally, the first REM burst lasts about 10 minutes, while the last may occur for over an hour or two. If you divide a sleep time of nine hours into three periods of three hours, the first third will be predominantly non-REM sleep and the last third will

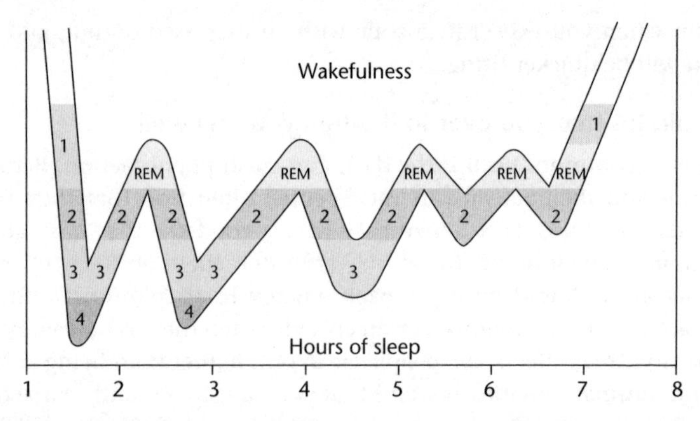

Figure 7.1 The sleep cycle through a night of sleep, showing rapid eye movement (REM) sleep and the four stages of non-REM sleep (1, 2, 3 and 4)

be mainly REM sleep. If one wakens from a full and good night's sleep it is usually from REM sleep or a short episode of stage 1 non-REM sleep, when you have a recollection of your last dream before it disappears as you grasp consciousness.

Stage 1 non-REM sleep occurs at the start and end of sleep and at potentially wakeful times during the night. It makes up about 5–10 per cent of total sleep time. It is characterized by twitches and occasional jerking movements. Sometimes one may experience what are called hypnagogic pseudo-hallucinations at this time, such as when one imagines falling off a gate and jerking awake. They are of no real significance. Stage 2 non-REM sleep, when one becomes less aware of the external environment, occurs throughout the sleep cycle and makes up about 40–50 per cent of sleep time. Stages 3 and 4 non-REM sleep occur mainly in the first third of the night and account for about 20 per cent of the sleep time. Sleep-walking seems to occur in this part of the sleep cycle. Stage 4 is the hardest sleep to be roused from. REM sleep makes up the remaining 20–25 per cent of the sleep time.

Even now we are not sure about the functions of the individual stages of sleep, but it seems that the whole process is essential to brain functioning and to the general health of the body. It is thought that non-REM sleep is associated with growth and repair of the brain and body and that REM sleep is associated with mental functions, dreaming and the processing of memory.

Broken sleep can therefore have quite an impact on how you feel. If you wake during non-REM sleep you may not have enough growth and repair sleep, which is important in rheumatic conditions, or you may not have enough REM and dream sleep, which can be important for your emotional health and your mood.

Obviously all the rheumatic problems can keep one awake or cause disturbed sleep, as can other conditions like anxiety, depression, an irritable bladder, prostate problems in men and so on. So too can habit problems, such as too much caffeine, tobacco or alcohol, or side effects from medication.

If you can, avoid taking sleeping tablets or tranquillizers. They need to be taken for only a week to develop a dependence on them. The Bach flower remedy, white chestnut – three or four drops in a small glass of water at night – may be all that you need to get off to sleep. It has no side effects. (See Chapter 8 for more about the Bach remedies.)

It could be emotional or a state of mind

People hate to think of anything being in the mind, as if it shows some sort of mental weakness. This is not the case. All people experience emotions and as a consequence think differently with differing emotions. If you are anxious it can affect sleep – you can be living on your nerves and be unable to relax. The consequence is tiredness.

If any negative emotion is present for too long it can eat away at you, drain you. Depression certainly does this, and people who are depressed commonly describe feeling apathetic, unable to motivate themselves and unable stop themselves from feeling tired. Correcting the emotional imbalance, the anxiety or the depression, can make a huge difference.

It could be fatigue rather than tiredness

Fatigue is different from simple tiredness. It seems to be more than just a matter of degree. Chronic fatigue syndrome can occur independently, but some people with arthritic and rheumatic conditions can experience very marked fatigue. Their energy levels seem to be permanently depleted and they are exhausted by the very slightest exertion. That exertion can be either physical or mental. This is quite common in fibromyalgia syndrome. It is poorly understood, but let me consider a few possible mechanisms that have been postulated.

Within each cell of the body there are tiny structures called mitochondria. The mitochondria are known to be the powerhouse of the body, because they are where a complex biochemical process called the Krebs cycle[7] takes place. Essentially, the body breaks down all the carbohydrates, fats and proteins into basic chemicals. These basic chemicals are transported to the mitochondria, where the Krebs cycle breaks them down into carbon dioxide, water and energy packets.

Glucose is the main chemical that is broken down in a series of eight steps, by being combined with other chemicals to cause it gradually to release its energy. These steps continue in a circular form that just goes on and on repeating itself. The energy is released as a chemical called adenosine triphosphate (ATP), which is transported to other parts of the cell where the energy is used to fuel all the other chemical processes of metabolism.

The Krebs cycle is an aerobic reaction, which means that it depends upon the presence of oxygen. If insufficient oxygen is present, an alternative method of producing energy is used. This is an anaerobic reaction, meaning that it takes place without oxygen. Instead of the readily disposable by-products of the Krebs cycle, this has lactate as a by-product. Lactate quickly chokes or stifles the process and it is hard to dispose of. The anaerobic reaction is far less efficient than the Krebs cycle and produces only a limited amount of energy.

This is what happens when muscles are over-used, as when running. The lactate that accumulates in the muscles produces painful cramp (or 'the burn'). Long-distance runners describe this as 'hitting the wall', in that all one's energy seems to have gone, the muscles just will not work and you literally cannot take another step.

In people who experience genuine fatigue, one of the theories is that their Krebs cycle stops working and they end up with the less efficient anaerobic reaction taking place, producing less energy and more lactate. Thus their muscles feel heavy, painful and stiff, and they just do not have enough energy for normal day-to-day functioning.

What can you do about it?

As I mentioned at the start of this chapter, unexplained tiredness needs investigation to find out whether it is being caused by the underlying problem, or by a new and as yet undiagnosed new condition, or as a side effect of medication. It is worth being analytical about your tiredness. Is it purely physical, or could it be to do with your emotions, your thinking, habits or your lifestyle? If you can spot it, chart it on the life cycle and you may see ways to change it.

For example, is it due to a problem of behaviour, such as the dash-and-crash effect? That is surely something that can be rectified. Or is it a sleep problem? If so, is it because of the physical condition, or an emotional state, or something in your lifestyle. Do you see what I mean?

You may need someone else to help you – a family member, partner, friend or health practitioner. Don't be afraid to ask for help.

Pacing yourself

This may seem an obvious thing to do, yet it is amazing how many people do not pace themselves. In fact, by simply learning how to pace yourself you can make a huge difference to your life. It is an extremely important part of self-help.

If you consider it, you do not have unlimited energy reserves; you can only do what your body allows. And as I suggested in the dash-and-crash phenomenon, many people experience the crash effect if they overdo things and use up more energy than they have available.

Start by getting an idea of how much you are currently doing. Keep a diary over a few days of everything you do and everything that seems to aggravate your symptoms. Just simply add up all the times you spend doing each activity. As you do so, score your energy levels out of 10, where 0 is no energy and 10 is bouncing with energy. See if a pattern develops. The dash-and-crash phenomenon will probably manifest itself and you will see the level beyond which you should not go.

There are three ways that you can effectively pace yourself. First, take adequate breaks. Secondly, split a task into two or three smaller tasks. For example, three trips carrying a lighter weight is easier than struggling with one large one. Finally, start by doing less than the level at which you know the dash-and-crash phenomenon will occur.

Tonics

Doctors used to use various tonics, but these are no longer considered to be effective and so cannot be prescribed. But, it is worth taking a multi-vitamin and mineral supplement to ensure that you are getting the recommended intake of vitamins, minerals and trace elements.

Apple cider vinegar and honey, marketed as Honegar is also a useful tonic. The dose is a dessertspoonful or two in water daily. Just be aware that it is acidic, so take care if you have a delicate stomach.

Noni juice is a drink prepared from a Hawaiian fruit. It is usually mixed with another fruit juice to improve its taste. I have taken this myself and felt that it did improve my energy levels while I was taking it. The dose is 30 millilitres a day, or about half a sherry glass.

Key points

- Do not assume that tiredness is due to your condition. Prolonged unexplained tiredness merits a medical opinion.
- Use the life cycle to try to pinpoint the tiredness and work out ways to improve it.
- Avoid sleeping tablets.
- Consider a multi-vitamin and mineral supplement.

8

Emotions and mind matters

'Take no notice of the disease, think only of the outlook on life of the one in distress,' 'said Dr Edward Bach. Our emotions alter the way we think. Human beings are not thinking machines. Our emotions make us what we are and modify our thoughts and are crucial to our sense of wellbeing.

Why we experience emotions at all is hard to explain. It is not as if they are learned in the same way that we learn facts and skills. The experience of anger is probably the same for a toddler living in the flatlands of Holland as it is for an old man who has lived his life in the foothills of the Himalayas. The things that trigger the anger in these people, however, may be very different.

Our emotions change our thought patterns. If you are angry about something you may well find your mind drifting to ways of venting that anger, possibly by getting even with someone or by making someone realize that you have been upset. That pattern of thought may be very different from the thoughts that come to you if you are feeling sad or anxious or guilty. And the thoughts you have when you are contented, happy or excited can be very different indeed.

There are many different theories about emotions. Some say that they are purely a result of thought and others suggest that they are a result of brain circuitry or the result of the body's chemistry and the way that chemistry affects the brain and the mind. It doesn't take long to get into chicken and egg arguments about emotions and thoughts, all of which is beyond the scope and space of a book such as this.

Yet as we saw in Chapter 5, on pain, emotions are intimately involved in the perception of chronic pain. We build up associations and we store up emotional memories. If we can release them or discharge them, there is a good chance of reducing some of the pain and symptoms associated with arthritis and rheumatism.

Negative emotions

It is the negative emotions that are likely to have an impact on someone with arthritis or rheumatism. In conventional practice only two such emotions are considered amenable to drug intervention – anxiety and depression. Both can be involved in arthritis and rheumatism and so are worth treating if they are detected. There are a range of antidepressants that may help and that can be prescribed by your doctor. As mentioned in Chapter 5, they may affect the threshold at which pain is perceived.

Hypericum, or St John's wort, is also a valuable treatment but is one that you should discuss with your doctor. Certainly, if you are taking any of the following drugs you should not take it at all: warfarin, ciclosporin, oral contraceptives, anticonvulsants, digoxin, theophylline or certain anti-HIV drugs. This is because St John's wort may reduce the effect of these drugs.

However, there are actually many negative emotions other than these two, and most of them also affect the person's emotional sphere, thereby also having an impact on the life cycle. For now I am going to cut to the quick and consider the amazing natural method of treatment of negative emotions devised by Dr Edward Bach. I am introducing them here because I believe them to be the simplest and one of the most effective means of dealing with many of these negative emotions. I have used them extensively throughout 30 years of medical practice.

The Bach flower remedies

Dr Edward Bach was a successful homoeopathic physician and bacteriologist attached to the Royal London Homoeopathic Hospital in the 1930s. As a research scientist he made several valuable contributions to homoeopathy. It was therefore a huge surprise to his colleagues when he gave up both his hospital appointments and his lucrative Harley Street practice in order to begin a search for the most simple and beneficial medicines amid the woods, fields and hedgerows of the English countryside.

It was Dr Bach's contention that people fell ill or failed to recover from illness because of their negative mental states. Using his research skills and his own highly developed intuition, he recorded 38 negative mental states, for each of which he discovered an antidote made from the flower of a wild plant, bush or tree.

Essentially he believed that the flowers of these plants had within them a signature, a positive energy pattern, which could redirect or neutralize a specific negative emotional state. Like a key, the correctly chosen remedy would unlock the corresponding negative emotional state.

Although they are often thought to be homoeopathic, they are in fact a unique form of therapy. The remedies are prepared directly from the plants and flowers to produce mother tinctures. Dr Bach divided them into seven groups according to the negative emotional states that they would relieve:

- Fear
- Uncertainty
- Insufficient interest in present circumstances
- Loneliness
- Over-sensitiveness to influences and ideas
- Despondency or despair
- Over-care for the welfare of others

For more details about individual remedies, see the Appendix.

Taking the Bach flower remedies

Stock bottles of the remedies can be obtained from chemists and health shops. A complete set of 38 is not necessary since most people can usually identify their temperament and negative emotions. Most people probably go through about five or six.

For temporary negative emotional states, take two drops of the appropriate stock remedy in a cup of water or fresh fruit juice. Take it three or four times a day until the emotion has settled.

Dr Bach also made a composite remedy called the rescue remedy. This is useful for dealing with the emotional effects of shock from any cause. It consists of:

- star of Bethlehem, for shock;
- rock rose, for terror and panic;
- impatiens, for tension and stress;
- cherry plum, for desperation; and
- clematis for feeling faint.

You can also mix up a bottle of your own, with up to six remedies. Success is greatest with a smaller number, I find. To make up your own bottle, add four drops of each remedy to a clean 30 millilitre bottle (which you can buy inexpensively from health shops or most supermarkets). Add about half a teaspoon of brandy as a preservative and top up with spring water. Just take this as you would a single remedy.

The beauty of the Bach flower remedies is that they are completely safe and can be taken at the same time as any drugs with no risk of interaction.

I really feel that these indications are worth studying and matching up with any of the negative emotions that you may have pinpointed in the life cycle. Or again, by studying this, you may find attitudes or tendencies that you had not put a name to before. Clearing these attitudes with these remedies may be one of the best things that you can do for your general wellbeing.

What sort of thoughts do you have?

That may sound a fairly banal question, for you will in the course of a day have many different types of thoughts. You will perhaps think about food, your appearance, your work, the various people in your life and so on. You may think about your state of health. If you have symptoms such as pain, stiffness and tiredness, they may make your condition a dominant part of your mental life. But what sort of thoughts are they? Are they helpful or unhelpful thoughts?

Unhelpful thoughts tend to be those with a negative connotation. Thoughts such as 'it is never going to get better!', 'no one has pain like me!', 'I can't cope any longer!' or 'somebody will have to do something!' are all unhelpful thoughts. Some of them may have their origin in your general outlook on life.

Before we go any further, get your exercise book out again and draw a series of lines and mark them from 0 to 10. Now score from 0 to 10 for each of these things:

- Pain. You will already have been keeping a pain diary, but let us consider it a little futher. Draw three separate lines for pain and score along it from 0 to 10, where 0 is no pain, 5 is moderate pain and 10 is the worst pain imaginable (perhaps like being burned in oil). Score first your least pain level, your average pain level and your worst pain level.
- Temper. A score of 0 is totally laid back, never angry; 10 is violent temper, flaring at the slightest thing.
- Jealousy.
- Holding a grudge.
- Patience or impatience.
- Optimism and pessimism. A score of 0 is always optimistic; 10 is totally pessimistic.

Do this now before you read on.

Your outlook and attitude

So what did you find? We are admittedly looking at different things here, but let's look at the pain readings. If your least readings are 0 or only 1 or 2 that is great. It shows that the condition can be controllable. If it is never less than a 5, that is at least moderate pain. If it is 7 or above that is severe pain most of the time. What about your readings at its worst – did you get up to 9 or 10? Did you even get beyond the scale? If you did, that means it is well-nigh unbearable pain – which it may well be, since it is you who is experiencing the pain.

But could it really be worse than being boiled in oil? Do you think so? A possible alternative explanation could be that you want to impress someone, yourself even, that it is unbearable.

What about temper? Are you sweetness and light? Do you never get cross, or are you volcanic? If you are 5 or above on average you may have an anger problem. But where does it come from? Is it because of your condition? If the condition was not so bad, would you be less irritable and less angry?

Or could it be possible that if you were less irritable and angry the condition would be easier to control?

How about jealousy? Is that an emotion that you can relate to?

And what about grudges? Do you always hold a grudge? Do you have to get even? Is it possible that you could be holding on to a symptom, just as you can hold on to a grudge?

Finally, on the optimism and pessimism score, are you at the extremes? To be an optimist certainly seems to be beneficial to people's general health. Optimistic people do seem to cope better with ailments, both mild and serious. On the other hand, pessimistic people fare less well. And so too do angry, hostile people. It simply is not good for you to hold on to negative emotions.

Now be clear about this: no judgement is meant in any of this. If you come out reading high on the anger, jealousy, grudge and pessimism scales, there may be real life reasons, legitimate logical reasons why you could feel as you do. But that does not mean that they are unalterable. It is possible that your outlook can be changed and that you can do it. Equally, it is very possible that the way you perceive symptoms can change or be eased by being able to let go a bit. And if you just take a little time to think about it, these emotions are mainly about 'holding on' to something. If you can stop holding on, and let go, those readings may drop and you may find that your coping levels with your condition improve considerably.

Helpful and unhelpful thinking

Let's go back to those few examples of thoughts that I gave. They are all examples of unhelpful thoughts. By that I mean that they do not help you. Take the first – 'it is never going to get better!' Well, how do you know? It may be the case, but a more helpful thought would be that 'it's pretty bad now, but I am sure it will get better.' The thing is that you do not know that it will not get better.

Or the second – 'no one has pain like me!' It is true, no one else experiences your pain, but it is probably incorrect to think that no one has pain that is worse than yours. It is not helpful to put yourself at the epicentre of the universe. This sounds like an extremely pessimistic thought, in that no one else can be as badly off. Don't think that, because it does not help you. A more helpful thought is that 'I am sure that other people have pains that are worse.'

Or the third example – 'I can't cope any longer!' That is worrying. Does it mean that you genuinely feel at rock bottom, depressed? If so you definitely need to seek help. And there is help available from your doctor. No one needs to feel so low. So what is so different about this moment, this time? It is not a time that is going to last. Let go of the thought and better, more cope-able times should be ahead. A helpful thought may be that you have managed, and that you have coped until now.

And finally – 'somebody will have to do something!' That smacks of anger, frustration. Who is that person who is going to have to do something? The doctor, the physiotherapist, your relative? Where do you come into the equation? How much are you going to help yourself? Again, it is accepted that someone else may have to do something, but don't approach it with anger. Let go of that and use a more helpful thought, such as, 'I must see how I can get someone to help me manage this.' It is you who is going to manage it, after all.

Challenging your thinking

OK, so it isn't easy to alter how you think. Not straight away at any rate. Yet it can be done. A good way is once again to use the life cycle concept, for which you will need the exercise book again. You used the grid in Table 8.1 before when we looked at pain. Draw it again, because now you are going to look at general symptoms. And also, you will be able to go back to the pain diary and fill in the questions column.

Table 8.1 Headings for each page of a diary of your general symptoms

Date	*Body*	*Emotions*	*Mind*	*Behaviour*	*Questions*

The idea is to keep a diary for a week. Any time that you become aware of a troublesome physical symptom, write it down at the time you have it in the *Body* section and score it from 1 to 10. Write how you were feeling at that time under *Emotions* and what you thought under *Mind*. Write what you were doing at that time and what you did to ease it. The important thing here is to do it at that moment, not later, when your perception of it may be different. It is the moment that you want to define.

The idea here is to build up a picture over a period of time of the pattern of symptoms, the level they are at and how you felt, thought and acted. After a week, look at the overall pattern and ask a few questions that will arise. These will relate to:

- How could you have felt differently?
- How could you have thought differently?
- What different action could you have taken?

Table 8.2

Date	*Body*	*Emotions*	*Mind*	*Behaviour*	*Questions*
29 September 2009	Headache 7/10 Neckache 7/10 Stiffness 6/10	Really depressed and scared that it will seize up completely one day	Here we go again. I knew I shouldn't have gardened yesterday! Life isn't worth it like this	Took pain killers.	

For example, suppose you have an arthritic neck and you experienced pain, stiffness and a headache in the morning. You might make the entries as shown in Table 8.2.

Looking at the pattern after a week, you may see a constant pattern in some areas. That should start making you question why is there a change. Why was a headache of level 5 one time and 7 another? Could it be because of differences in the mood, the thinking, the behaviour?

And the questions you can start to ask are, for example, 'was the pain really a 7?' Could it have been a 5, and if so did you need to take a pain-killer when the level was only a 5? Think about how you could change the ways that you were thinking, by asking yourself questions about alternative helpful thoughts rather than the unhelpful ones that you had.

Follow this line and you will see that there is scope for change and scope for improvement in the scores. And that means improved coping.

You can become more optimistic

If you are of a pessimistic disposition it is possible that you may have a harder time with arthritis and rheumatism than an optimistic person will. Not only that, but there is good evidence that optimists are less likely to experience depression, stress and anxiety. They also have fewer colds, are less likely to have heart trouble, and live longer. It seems that pessimism adversely affects one's immune system. And finally, some studies have shown that pessimistic people are more accident-prone.

Now a pessimist might say, 'Of course, that will be me, it always happens to me.'

But it doesn't, in fact. These things may happen not because someone is unluckier, or actually accident-prone. It happens because a person's outlook on life can create a behaviour that is likely to be self-determining. If you expect bad things to happen, you may be more likely to do things that make them occur.

Logotherapy

I first came across the works of Viktor Frankl at the start of my career, when I was working in psychiatry. Frankl was a Holocaust survivor and the founder of a system of psychiatry known as logotherapy. This is sometimes referred to as the 'Third Viennese School of Psychiatry' (Sigmund Freud's being the first and Alfred Adler's the second). Frankl developed his theories during stays in three different concentration camps, including the dreaded Auschwitz. His parents and his wife all died in the dreadful conditions of the camps, yet he survived because he made it his aim to help others to survive by altering the way they thought. He clearly saved many people from suicide.

In establishing his philosophy of logotherapy, Frankl established three basic beliefs:

1 That life has meaning in all circumstances, even the most miserable ones.
2 That our main motivation is our will to find meaning in life.
3 That we have freedom to find meaning in what we do and in what we experience.

The essence of all this is that we have choice as to how we view things. One must work against a tendency to be pessimistic and endeavour to become an optimist.

Self-talk

Self-talk is the name that we give to the endless stream of thoughts that run through our heads every day. Pessimists, who may be more prone to depression, tend to have many negative automatic thoughts. Let me give you four examples. These may be quite foreign to optimists:

- Pessimists magnify and filter – that is, they magnify the negative factors in a situation and filter out the positives. For example, a pessimist might complete ten tasks very well in a day, but one does not go so well. That one task is the one that preoccupies the pessimist, while the others are filtered out and forgotten.
- Pessimists personalize everything. A bad event is assumed to be their fault, because of something they may have done, or because someone has reacted against them.
- Pessimists catastrophize everything. They only see the worst scenario. Because of this they may adopt an avoidance behaviour.
- Pessimists only see in black or white, never in shades of grey. It is good or bad, more often bad than good.

But it can be changed. To do so you have to develop that self-awareness that I have talked about. You should be aware of the self-talk thought dialogue that takes place in your mind, but stop listening to the negative side. Just because bad things may have happened in the past does not mean that is how the future will be. The past is not the same as the future and there is no reason why it should be unless you allow it to be. Use your mind. Instead of thinking 'I can't do this', think 'this is an opportunity to do well.' Don't think 'I haven't time to do this'; instead think 'I'm going to make time.' And instead of 'it always happens to me', tell yourself, 'there is no reason it will happen to me'.

Letting go

Negative emotions, such as hate, guilt and anger, eat away at you. They are of no value to you, so should not be nurtured. Now believe me, many people do nurture negative emotions. They harbour ill-will, they plot about getting even with someone or some organization, but without any benefit. All they do is perpetuate negativity in their whole life cycle. It is small wonder that pains persist, stiffness won't go and people feel so tired. Holding on to emotions means holding on to thought patterns, engenders associations within the brain and the pain matrix, and uses up a lot of energy.

Now of course that isn't the whole story, but it may be part of the story. Self-awareness, if you are truthful with yourself, will reveal it. You have to let it go. But how?

Well, good old-fashioned forgiveness is one thing. Say it, keep saying it to yourself and eventually you will let it go and it will stop harming you.

People hold on to anger about perceived injustice. This often happens in litigation situations. The problem there is that there may be an unconscious mechanism that keeps hold of a symptom until the case is won! Yet that doesn't always occur and the pain matrix gets stuck, and hence chronic pain develops.

Imagine some people who have run up against an insurance problem. They get cross with the insurance firm and feel determined to get the better of the firm. They phone and phone, demanding to go ever higher up the ladder. And they spend hours working out how they are going to make the firm sorry that they crossed swords in the first place. The truth is that the organization does not feel anything. It is composed of people who are just doing their job. They will not be hurt, so hostility is wasted effort. The grudge is wasted emotion.

Let go of grudges, lose the hostility and give yourself a chance to be less stiff and more supple.

You can try adding this exercise to your relaxation and imagination sessions. Identify the emotion, focus on it and imagine that you are like the giant Gulliver tied down by a series of little threads. None of them is very strong in itself, but when there are lots they tie you down. Imagine that your mind is going round and snipping them one at a time. Feel that release as you let it go. Keep repeating that and you will find that, surprisingly, it can help to let go.

Consider the words you use

You may already have noticed that when recording how you feel you have used certain adjectives. They are a normal part of speech. Indeed, when talking about how you feel you may use exactly the same words. For example, in talking about pain do you ever use words or expressions such as 'excruciating', 'agonizing', 'back-breaking', 'killing', 'unbearable', 'unending', 'unendurable'? Or any number of worse and unprintable words?

They all conjure up unpleasant images. And those images may indeed be how it feels, yet if you think about it you see how very negative they are. Indeed, the words that you use can also chain you into a negative manner of thinking about your symptoms. It is worth modifying the words by bringing them down a degree or two. Make them less negative. Rather than 'excruciating' and so on, try thinking of 'uncomfortable', 'sore', 'achy'.

And you might try and use the word 'discomfort' instead of pain.

This isn't in any way an attempt to belittle your symptoms. Think about how you describe hunger for a moment. Everyone gets hungry, but do you use the words 'starving', 'ravenous' or 'famished'? If you do, is that actually correct?

The point is that inappropriate wording reinforces a thought. When you use a word to emphasize to other people how you are feeling, you reinforce the thought in your own mind. Similarly, you can use your mind to lessen the intensity or the importance of a symptom.

Distraction

Distraction is an extremely good method of easing unhelpful thoughts. Music, a hobby, an activity or an interest can all take your mind off things. So too can being with fun people, relatives and friends.

And using and appreciating all your senses can help. It has been shown that literally smelling the flowers can induce mood enhancement. So make an effort to appreciate everything that you see, hear and do.

Auto-suggestion

Émile Coué was a French psychologist and pharmacist who developed the concept of auto-suggestion. Put very simply it is the use of a mantra-like phrase, such as 'every day in every way I am getting better and better'. By repeating this to yourself several times at the start and the end of the day, when you focus on just these words, you can begin to develop a positive way of thinking. It is a simple thing to do and is really worth trying.

It is also worth using various affirmations. Write them down and paste them on your computer, on your bathroom mirror and in your wallet or purse. They act as little positive reminders. Things like:

- 'I am in control.'
- 'It is always possible.'
- 'I create the circumstances; the circumstances do not create me.'

And you may be surprised at how much they will help.

Key points

- The Bach flower remedies are an excellent way of releasing negative emotions.
- Avoid unhelpful thinking.
- Challenge your thoughts.
- Strive to be an optimist – there is positive in everything.

9

What can I do to help myself?

We come now to the final two spheres of the life cycle model. These relate to your behaviour and your lifestyle. Clearly these two spheres are very much inter-related.

By 'behaviour', I mean actions and reactions. It is the way that you do things, whether consciously or unconsciously. It includes your eating habits, your exercise levels, your social habits and the ways that you act because of your health.

By 'lifestyle', I mean your work, leisure pursuits, relationships, and all the events that have an impact on your overall wellbeing. This can include financial concerns, family and relative matters, the overall pace of your life, and the demands that may be placed upon you or that you place on yourself and upon others.

Unhelpful behaviour

It is important to consider any habit that you may have come to depend on that may be affecting you adversely.

Smoking

Top of the list is smoking. People smoke for different reasons and many confirmed addicts genuinely feel that it is their only pleasure. You have to question this, because it is usually the addiction that is speaking. It is not so much that it is pleasurable, but that doing without it produces unpleasant symptoms and feelings.

The fact is that smoking does not help your body in any way. When you light tobacco and start smoking a cigarette, pipe or cigar, you are potentially taking about 300 undesirable chemicals into your system. As you get half-way down the cigarette, the intense heat and further chemical degradation increases that number to over 1500 chemicals, most of which are toxic. Giving up smoking is one of the best things that you can do.

There is ample evidence that smoking is harmful to people with rheumatic conditions and that the risk of developing rheumatoid arthritis is doubled if you smoke.[8] It certainly has been demonstrated to make fibromyalgia symptoms worse.[9]

Your doctor can direct you to a smoking cessation clinic or prescribe various agents that can help. In addition, acupuncture and hypnotherapy are other options that have demonstrated success.

Alcohol

In contrast to smoking, drinking some alcohol can be helpful to your wellbeing, but excessive drinking or binge drinking can definitely be unhelpful.

It is currently recommended that men should drink no more than 21 units of alcohol a week and no more than four units in any 24 hours. Women should drink no more than 14 units a week and no more than three units in any 24 hours. A unit is 8 grams by weight of alcohol, which equates to a half pint of (4 per cent) beer or lager, a pub measure of a spirit or sherry, or a small glass of wine. No need to cut it out, just don't go over the limit!

Obesity

Being overweight has an obvious effect on the joints and the whole locomotor system. But it is bad for the whole body, including the heart. Do not fall into believing that fat tissue is biologically inactive, for it is not. It does produce a hormonal effect, as is shown in its tendency to worsen the prognosis of various hormonally dependent cancers.

There may be difficulty in losing weight because of a tendency to be less active, yet it is desirable to stay as trim as possible and not find that your weight is gradually increasing.

Inactivity

Inactivity may be linked to being overweight, and it may of course be true that your condition can limit the amount of exercise you can do. Yet inactivity is not good for anyone with arthritis and rheumatism, and you should try to be as active as your condition permits.

On the other hand it is important to be careful if your joints are actively inflamed. Over-activity of an inflamed joint can result in further damage, so during active inflammation the joint needs to be protected. Here you must ignore the oft-repeated advice 'no gain without pain.' In the case of joints, the pain should not be ignored and you should definitely pace yourself.

Helpful behaviour

All the things you put into practice from your reading of this book should encourage helpful behaviour.

Good nutrition

I am going to talk at greater length about this in Chapter 11. There is a great deal that you can do to help yourself by eating a good wholesome diet that is not excessive to your needs. For a lot of people with rheumatic conditions, cutting out certain foods may be crucial.

Exercise within your limits

The benefits of exercise are well established. Exercise helps your body to maintain the function of all your organs and systems, including the brain. The locomotor system benefits from regular use. Immobility will result in loss of muscle bulk, the bones will lose calcium and fibrous tissue will become less flexible, all of which will add to the seeming progression of the condition.

You may have limited mobility as a result of your condition, but it is important to be as active as you can.

Being sociable

It is important to maintain your social networks with family, friends and workmates. One of the problems that can occur with rheumatic conditions is their tendency to make you isolated. This is to be avoided at all costs.

So what do I mean by isolation? People who experience unrelieved pain from arthritis or rheumatism over a considerable period of time often feel trapped and helpless. When their condition is first diagnosed they may have been told that their condition is not curable and that they will have to live with it and control it as best they can. Pain-killers and some form of anti-inflammatory drug may have helped, but in some people they provoke anxiety because they may find that they need to be taken regularly. This tends to make one think that the condition is progressing.

Often a vicious circle develops, which keeps them anchored to their pain. It may seem to them that friends and family just don't understand the pain that they are experiencing. This can make them withdraw into themselves, sink into depression and start to feel isolated. Because they feel isolated they spend more time thinking about the pain, which causes fear and despair. This fear can take many forms. For example, it can be fear that they will never get better, fear that it is going to deteriorate rapidly and fear about earning a living. The effect of this fear is to intensify the tension, depress the spirits and increase the feeling of isolation. When this happens the mind focuses back on the pain, with the result that the pain is reinforced.

And when you look at this in terms of the life cycle you can see the interaction of all these spheres, and the end-result is a lifestyle change and isolation. It is this that can make the condition worse, so it is all the more important to keep up your friends and acquaintances and avoid isolating yourself.

Other people's behaviour

Other people's behaviour can be an important issue. The behaviour of friends and relatives can sometimes make your condition worse! You may never have considered this, but it may be true.

When people see that you are struggling they may take certain aspects of your life over. They may do various tasks for you because they feel that they are sparing you the effort. The thing is that when they do this they are effectively rewarding you for having a condition. This can have a subtle psychological effect, since we respond to rewards by reinforcing our behaviour. Thus, they may be enhancing the condition.

It is worth analysing this, so get your exercise book out again and look at all the things that people do for you. For example, are you spared from shopping, doing dishes, carrying shopping? Look at everything and look at the things that you are 'not allowed' to do. The question is, could you do them?

If you think the answer is yes to any of them you may be able to alter the other person's behaviour, by persuading him or her that it may be good for you to try the activity. And if you cannot manage that activity in one go, split it up into several stages. That is back to pacing, of course.

You may worry that you will offend the other person by asking this, but you can modify the behaviour by permitting the person to help you to manage that activity. For example, it is better to try to go shopping with help than to have it done for you. The point is that sometimes people take over an activity, which can deprive you of your independence. It is a vicious circle, because the reinforcing of your behaviour reinforces the other person's behaviour and keeps you at the reduced level of functioning.

Get to know the pattern of your problem

It is worth taking a few days to monitor the pattern of your condition. This was shown by a study of people with osteoarthritis of the hands, who were monitored over a ten-day period. They were asked to monitor their pain and stiffness levels at six specific times of the day: on waking, at bedtime and every four hours in between. In addition, they were asked to perform a manual dexterity test each time they rated their pain and stiffness. This was a timed test in which they had to pass a number of objects through a tube into a container. If any were dropped, they had to start again, so that they achieved a measurable score each time they did the test.

It was found that for 75 per cent of the participants pain and stiffness were worst in the morning and at bedtime. Mid-afternoon was the best time. More specifically, pain was least between lunchtime and 6.00 p.m., whereas stiffness was least between 3.00 p.m. and teatime. Manual dexterity was best when pain and stiffness scores were at their least, which for most people was at about 4.00 p.m.

This little exercise is worth doing in order to gauge the pattern or the rhythm of your condition. If you can do that you can actually plan your day a bit better. For example, performing a manual task after teatime may be the worst time for you, since your pain levels may be rising, as might your stiffness. The further activity may make the pain worse.

So, get out your exercise book again and do this little test over ten days, using the score of 0 to 10 for pain and stiffness. I will leave you to think up a suitable dexterity test to do yourself over one minute.

Choose your exercise

People often reduce their activities when they develop arthritis or rheumatism. This is understandable, but it is the wrong thing to do. Exercise keeps joints and muscles mobile. You also maintain the circulation to them, so that they get the nutrients they need delivered to them and the waste products are taken away.

Exercise is good, except when joints are acutely inflamed. Joint protection is vital, as we shall see in the next section (see page 80).

There are three types of exercise that you should know about. All are important, but you have to work within your capabilities. And you should schedule exercise carefully after working out the pattern of your pain and stiffness, as I mentioned above.

1 Range-of-movement exercises are gentle stretching exercises to maintain the suppleness of the joints through their range of movement. They should be done each day for five repetitions of each one. There is nothing mysterious in these; they simply involve using the joints. For example, to exercise the neck, while sitting in a chair, try

touching your right shoulder with your right ear, and then do the same to the left. Do it five times each side. Then, starting with the head in a neutral position, turn the head as if you were to look over your right shoulder. Then gently turn it to the left as if to look over your left shoulder. Do this five times in each direction. Finally, start with your chin on your chest and slowly tip your head as far back as you can, without feeling dizzy, and then lower it back to your chest. Do five repetitions of each of these exercises.

And you simply go through the range of movements with your shoulders, elbows, wrists, hips, knees and ankles.

2 Strengthening exercises are used to improve the muscles' strength in order to make the muscles around the joints as strong as possible, so that pain will be reduced. It really will help. There are two types of strengthening exercise – isometric and isotonic. In isometric exercises, the muscles are tightened without moving the joint – for example, holding one wrist and trying to flex the biceps muscle at the same time against the resistance you have produced. In isotonic exercises, you strengthen the muscles by moving the joint – for example, by lifting weights. However, make sure that you do not overdo it with the weights. It is worth getting advice and having a fitness programme worked out with a professional fitness coach. These isometric and isotonic strengthening exercises should be done two or three times a week.
3 Endurance exercises speed up the heart and improve breathing. These are done for 20 minutes at a time, ideally three times a week.

Everyone with arthritis and rheumatism should be trying to do the first two types regularly. The third type should be planned with your doctor, physiotherapist or fitness coach, and what you do will depend upon the severity of your condition.

It is a good idea to talk exercising over with your doctor in the first instance and to make a plan or a program of exercises. Ideally, you want to include all three types of exercise in your plan. The limiting factors may be the type of problem you have, the presence of inflammation, the degree of joint stability or instability, the presence of artificial joints and your general level of health.

Good exercises

Good exercises for people with arthritis and rheumatism include:

- Walking – good for mobility and locomotor system health.
- Yoga – good for maintaining posture, suppleness and relaxation.

- Tai chi – a gentle Chinese martial art, excellent for using gentle movements through the range of movements; also good discipline and good for balance.
- Swimming – a non-weight bearing exercise, good for stamina, strength and suppleness. Just take care in choosing the right stroke. The breast stroke may not be good for people with neck and knee arthritis.
- Cycling – good non-weight bearing, two-sided exercise.
- Jogging – good exercise that should not do harm since running is a natural movement, as long as the individual is fit enough. Run on grass to reduce hard impact.

In working out your exercise program you need to aim at the following:

- Stick to the plan as much as you can
- Build up gradually
- Don't overdo it – remember to pace yourself
- Stop if your body tells you to – in other words, pain induced by exercise should be listened to
- Don't exercise a hot, inflamed joint
- Establish realistic goals – learn to crawl before you walk before you run!
- Work with your exercise adviser

Joint protection

The purpose of joint protection is to reduce strain on joints, minimize pain and prevent joint damage. It is something that anyone with arthritis must keep in mind and build into their lifestyle.

This is an area where your occupational therapy department can help immeasurably, so it is worth seeking their advice. An appointment at a hospital department can be arranged through the rheumatology clinic or your rheumatology specialist nurse, and if necessary a home appointment to assess your needs may be possible.

The principles of joint protection are fairly simple and a matter of common sense.

1. Respect pain. If you have more pain two hours after exercise than you had before, you have done too much. You need to reduce the level next time.
2. Avoid activities that cause joint pain. This means that you should be prepared to use tools, like bottle openers and jar openers, if needs be. Similarly, if standing at a sink causes back pain, consider sitting to do the task, or do it in little stages.

3 Avoid actions that will encourage joint deformity. Take advice about appropriate aids and adaptations. There are all sorts of equipment on offer, such as long-handled spoons, raised toilet seats, handles on baths and so on. The Disabled Living Foundation offers free advice and factsheets on these (see Useful addresses at the end of the book). It is also worth learning to do things with both sides of the body to take the load off a particular joint or limb, such as turning on a tap with one hand and turning it off with the other. Try to avoid using a pincer grip between finger and thumb when lifting things with the hands. Using the palm to carry things is less likely to cause damage to finger joints.
4 Always try to use larger and stronger muscles. For example, use both arms when carrying something. Don't depend on a single, smaller joint, especially a joint of the hands.
5 Strive for the best posture you can, but try to avoid static positions and immobility.
6 Balance activity with rest to conserve energy.
7 Try to keep your weight down, for being overweight can throw extra pressure on joints.
8 Consider using a cushion to support joints when in bed. This is particularly the case with arthritic knees. A cushion between the knees may take the pressure of one joint off the other when lying on one's side.

Good posture

Good posture is something that you really should strive for, and work on. The straighter you are, the better you will be able to protect your joints. The problem with so many of these conditions is that they cause discomfort. The body automatically gets into the position of least discomfort, which is often not the best position. Indeed, after a period of time the muscles retain a memory to keep you in that position. Thus, pain, stiffness and some degree of tiredness will result.

Once again, self-awareness is important. Stand and look in a full length mirror. Without trying to correct your posture, just observe. Start with your shoulders. Is one higher than the other? Is your neck turned or twisted? Is your head lop-sided? And your chest, is one side of it turned more to the fore than the other? The way your clothes hang will give you clues. If you lift your shirt or blouse, is your tummy button facing directly forward or is it pointing to the side? And your pelvis, is it rotated? Now look at your feet. Is one in front of the other? If so, it may be because you have rotated your pelvis.

If you turn to the side, how are your curves? A healthy back has three natural curves: a slight forward curve in the neck (the cervical curve), a slight backward curve in the upper back (the thoracic curve), and a slight forward curve in the low back (the lumbar curve). Good posture means keeping these three curves in balanced alignment.

Strong and flexible muscles also are essential to good posture. Abdominal, hip, and leg muscles should all be kept as well toned as possible to support your back's natural curves. And of course, your hips, knees and ankles balance your back's natural curves when you move, making it possible to maintain good posture in any position.

You can check the three curves of your spine quite easily. Stand with your back to a wall, heels about three inches from the wall. Place one hand behind your neck, with the back of the hand against the wall, and the other hand behind your low back with the palm against the wall. If there is excessive space between your back and the wall, such that you can easily move your hands forward and back more than one inch, some adjustment in your posture may be necessary to restore the normal curves of your spine.

Sitting positions can cause problems, and are worth focusing on when working. Sit with your back firmly against a chair, making sure that the chair is low enough to allow both feet to be placed on the floor, ideally with the knees slightly higher than the hips. Keep your head up and avoid leaning forward. If you work long hours at a desk or word processor, keep your chair close in to the desk to help maintain your upright position.

Yoga and the Alexander technique can both help arthritis and rheumatism. A recent small study from the University of California[10] found that when a group of elderly people did yoga for six months they saw a decrease in the upper spine curve of 5 per cent, as opposed to no change in those who did no yoga. Effectively it reduced the excessive curve that results in the 'dowager's hump' that is so commonly seen in people with osteoporosis.

Heat and cold

Opinion is divided among health professionals about the relative merits or otherwise of heat and cold treatments. My own view is that both are very valuable, but the way they work depends upon the individual person: the person's experience is the determining factor. Some people will benefit from heat and not cold, and vice versa.

Having said this, I think that the following are good rules of thumb:

- Cold packs numb sore areas and will reduce inflammation. The numbness increases the threshold at which pain is felt.
- Moist heat is good for pain in some people. If you are one of these people you will probably experience ease in a hot shower or a hot bath.
- Some people fare better when heat is alternated with cold. For example, a warm wheat pack is applied to a painful part for five minutes, replaced with a cold pack (a pack of frozen vegetables applied through a towel) for five minutes, which is then replaced by the heat for a further five minutes before going back to cold and finally heat again. It really is an individual choice.
- Cold seems to be most effective when applied to a painful area within 48 hours of the onset of the pain.
- Heat seems to be more effective when applied to an area that has remained painful for longer than 48 hours.

Daily living equipment

In order to protect joints and just to make life easier, you may consider using an aid of some sort. Many people do not like the idea of this, since they think that it will show that their condition is getting the better of them. This is not the case. Human beings are intelligent creatures and are distinguished from most other mammals by being tool-users. We all use tools in daily work and life, whether they are hammers, forceps, knitting needles or laptops. Daily living equipment includes all sorts of aids, or tools, which can be used to help you do tasks that have started to become difficult as a result of a medical condition.

There are four types of daily living equipment:

1 Items for people with a significant disability to help them overcome a particular difficulty, such as a wheelchair, mobility aids, a bath board or a raised toilet seat.
2 Standard equipment, or labour-saving devices that can be used to ease the effort of a particular task, such as a food processor that removes the need to chop vegetables, an electric tin-opener instead of a manual one, a vacuum cleaner.
3 Standard equipment that has been modified, such as a long-handled hairbrush or comb, long-handled spoons or special grips for cutlery for those who have difficulty holding utensils.
4 Custom-made equipment for the individual to overcome a problem that is unique to that person.

Walking sticks and mobility aids

These really can make a difference, provided you get the right one for you and use it properly. Your occupational therapist or physiotherapist will be able to advise you.

Take someone with osteoarthritis of the hip. A walking stick will take 13.5 kg of his or her weight, which can be a significant reduction of the force on the joint whenever they walk.

A standard wooden walking stick or cane has a curved handle, which is useful for hooking onto one's arm to free you to do some manual task. Lightweight aluminium ones are more robust and their length can be adjusted. A bariatric walking stick (Figure 9.1A) is a heavy-duty one, usually made of metal with a curved neck so designed to distribute the walker's weight directly over the handle. It is useful for larger people, up to a weight of about 225 kilograms (35 stone).

The handle of any walking stick needs to be comfortable and of the right size. A curved handle can make matters worse in someone with arthritis of the hands, since it concentrates pressure on to a small area at the base of the palm. A Fischer handle (Figure 9.1B) is a specially moulded plastic handle, which may be best for someone with arthritis of the hands.

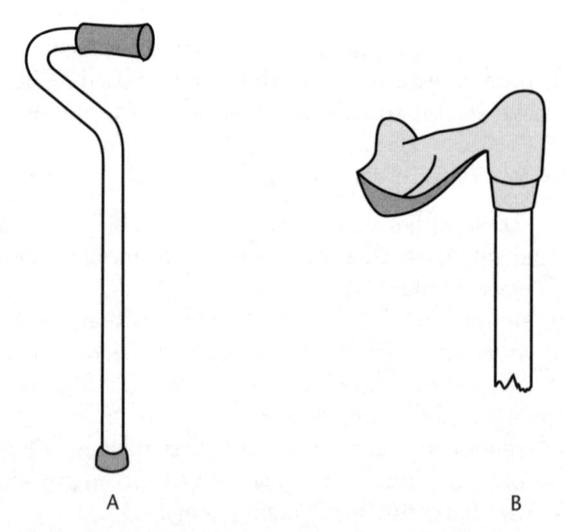

Figure 9.1A. A bariatric walking stick with a curved neck B. A walking stick with a Fischer handle

The length of the stick is crucial. As a rule of thumb, the right length is such that the length from the top of the handle to the tip of the stick is the same as the distance from the wrist crease to the floor. Thus, when standing erect in everyday shoes, holding the stick still, the elbow will bend to about 15 degrees. This allows good extension of the stick when walking and will help in weightbearing.

Always make sure that the stick has a good rubber ferrule on the bottom that will give a good grip.

Finally, use the stick the right way. If you have an arthritic right hip, use the stick on the left side; otherwise you just hobble and will not achieve the ease that you need.

Tripods and tetrapods are pyramid sticks with three or four legs. They may be helpful for a person who has a balance problem. And where balance is a real issue, a Zimmer frame may be an option to discuss with your occupational therapist.

Wheelchairs

There are different types of wheelchair. The commonest ones are attendant (push) wheelchairs and self-propelled wheelchairs. Powered wheelchairs, of which there are four types, are also available.

If a wheelchair is necessary, you certainly need advice from your doctor or occupational therapist, who can refer you to the NHS Wheelchair Service, who can make an assessment of your needs and discuss funding options, if you are deemed eligible. There are variations according to local referral methods, since some areas operate a self-referral system. You can check your local situation on <www.wheelchairmanagers.nhs.uk/services.asp>.

Sex

Arthritis and rheumatism can affect this special part of life, and may strain relationships. Once again, you can look at this in terms of the life cycle model, thinking of it in terms of body, emotions, thoughts, behaviour, lifestyle and relationship. For example, at the body level there may be pain and discomfort in certain positions. At the emotional level people may feel conscious about how they look if they perceive that their joints have become ungainly or unattractive. Fears of being unattractive can lead to avoiding the physical side of a relationship, which in turn can make a partner back off.

If there is a developing issue, it is worth sitting down and having an honest discussion about feelings and loving. You may want to consider outside help in the form of counselling, which your doctor can arrange. There really is no need to be embarrassed about this.

Some sexual positions are more comfortable than others and it is worth exploring and discussing. And being prepared, by being relaxed, is so important. Try a relaxing bath beforehand, so that the muscles and joints are more comfortable. Similarly, there is no harm in taking a pain-killer. And do not rush. Take your time and enjoy the process of loving one another.

Key points

- Avoid habits that are harmful.
- Keep yourself as trim as you can. It is useful to monitor your weight, so weigh yourself every day – a good time is the morning, before breakfast, either undressed or with night clothes only.
- Make exercise part of your life – range-of-movement exercises, strengthening exercises and, if able, endurance exercise.
- Observe the rhythm of your condition.
- Work on your posture.
- Consider daily living equipment.

10

Home, work and benefits

By now you will have identified a great deal about how your condition is affecting all the spheres of your life. Indeed, I hope that you will have started to devise strategies yourself to deal with some of the issues that you have identified in each sphere.

Home

I have already touched on some of the daily living equipment that you can access in order to ease tasks, thereby lessening strain and conserving your energy. Once again it is worth getting your exercise book out and thinking about all the things that you do in the home and then charting those things that cause you difficulty. Identification is the key and you can look at goals and strategies to achieve those goals.

For example, you may think about cleaning the house. What causes the most difficulty? Is it the fact that you like to get it all done at once? It is worth taking it apart like this:

- Plan when you are going to do it according to the rhythm of your condition, as discussed in Chapter 9.
- Plan it so that you can conserve energy. Don't be dashing about all over the place, but aim at doing one area at a time.
- Prioritize what needs doing and be prepared to leave the non-essential things until another time.
- Break tasks down. Tasks do not need to be completed in one go. For example, if you have difficulty carrying, don't carry wet clothes, wait for them to dry. Stage the processes.
- Grade tasks according to whether they are light, medium or heavy. You do that by judging how much energy you will expend, and how much difficulty they will cause.
- Pace yourself and take a break in between tasks. Certainly do not do two heavy tasks one after the other.
- Have rest places about the house. Invest in extra stools so that you can rest between tasks and also consider sitting and doing things rather than standing. Do you really need to stand at the sink? Can you sit while you prepare food?

- Use daily living equipment if needed. But also consider the way that you do things. Use scissors rather than ripping open packs or bags. Use an electric whisk rather than a hand one.
- Think: identification of problem, strategy.

Work and ergonomics

People work for many reasons. Work can give you self esteem, financial security, comradeship and a host of other things. Your condition may start to cause you difficulties at work and it is again worth looking at all the things that you do at work and identifying problems in order to work out appropriate strategies.

Your occupational therapist or the occupational health department at work may be able to help by looking at the ergonomics of your work. Ergonomics is the science of making the job, occupation and workplace right for the individual, to minimize strain during the work and to maintain health and, of course, productivity.

For example, a computer operator should have the screen at an appropriate viewing distance and appropriate viewing angle to avoid eye strain and neckache. The seat or chair should allow the posture to be maintained to support the back, allow a sitting or seat back angle of 90 degrees and a knee bend angle of 90 degrees. There should be an adequate keyboard so that the wrists can be kept straight and the elbow angle at 90 degrees.

And for people who stand a lot, there should be similar considerations for posture, adequate sitting if it is feasible, and proper rests.

Benefits

It may be, of course that your condition is such that you are having difficulty with work. If you are unable to work at all you may be eligible for Disability Living Allowance (DLA). This is a tax-free benefit for adults over the age of 16 and under the age of 65 years who need help with personal care or walking. You can get this whether or not you work.

The DLA has two components – a care component, if you need help to look after yourself, and a mobility component, if you have difficulty walking. You can qualify for one component or both. There are currently three weekly rates for the care component of the DLA: a lower rate of £18.65, a middle rate of £47.10 and the highest rate of £70.35. There are currently two weekly rates for the mobility component of the

DLA: a lower rate of £18.65 and a higher rate of £49.10. Your individual circumstances affect the amount that you are paid.

If you are over 65 years of age you may be eligible to receive Attendance Allowance. To be eligible you have to demonstrate difficulty in looking after yourself in areas such as washing and bathing, dressing, eating and going to the toilet. There are two weekly rates for the Attendance Allowance: a lower rate of £47.10 and a higher rate of £70.35.

You can apply for these allowances directly online at <www.direct.gov.uk>, or you can obtain a pack by phoning the Benefit Enquiry line – see Useful addresses at the end of the book. Alternatively, you can seek advice from your local Jobcentre Plus office or your local social security office.

You may or may not need a medical examination. If you find that you are eligible and you are successful in obtaining the DLA or the Attendance Allowance, it might increase other benefits, such as Income Support, Housing benefit and Working Tax Credit.

Motability

The Motability Scheme enables disabled people to exchange either their higher-rate mobility component of the DLA or their War Pensioners' Mobility Supplement to obtain a new car, a powered wheelchair or a scooter.

11

Diet – one man's meat is another man's poison

Diet cures more than the lancet, as Miguel de Cervantes says in *Don Quixote*. It has been my experience that about 50 per cent of people with arthritic and rheumatic conditions can be helped to some degree by dietary change. Over the years I have looked at and tried out several of the diets that have been advocated and have come to the conclusion that no one diet that will help everyone, but that it is certainly worth trying some of the diets for a six-week period. At the very least, if you can identify foods that are doing you harm or which make your symptoms worse, you can exclude them.

In this chapter I run through a few of the dietary changes that I have found useful and look at foods and supplements that may be worth taking because they are anti-inflammatory in action.

Diets

First of all, what is a diet? That might sound a banal question, but most people misunderstand the meaning of the word. A diet is not just something that you do to lose weight. A diet means the foods that you regularly consume. Everyone is therefore on a diet.

Yet being overweight is something you should definitely try to avoid if you have arthritis or rheumatism. The less weight your joints have to bear and the less weight that your muscles have to move, the more efficiently they can function.

I am not going to spend long on the topic of weight control, because if you can get on a diet that is right for you – and by that I mean one on which you seem to function best and your symptoms are less severe – you will probably find that your weight comes down and remains stable. You should aim for a Body Mass Index[11] of 25. If you are aiming to bring your weight down, make it a long term goal to get to 25, and choose slow and realistic targets on the way.

You can of course count calories and apply the model of the second law of thermodynamics, which many doctors quote at people. Very simply, this means that if the energy intake exceeds the energy output, the energy will be stored. This basically means that it will be stored as fat. It is, of course, very hard to work out what you have taken in and even harder to work out how much energy you have used up.

I am all in favour of simple rules of thumb and I am a great believer in using what has been described as nature's food bowl. The theory is that your cupped hands should give you the measure of food that you should take at any meal. Don't heap it too highly, but that is the quantity of food that should be allowed on your plate at any of the three meals. Add in the additional rules of thumb that you don't go back for seconds and you should never rise from the table feeling full, and you avoid the unhealthy habit of 'eating up'.

Elimination diet

An elimination diet is not a dietary change to stay on, but is simply a diet to go on in order to identify any foods to which you may be sensitive and which could be provoking your condition. Essentially, it's a very restrictive diet containing only foods unlikely to provoke a reaction. It demands willpower and strict discipline. If you are on any medication, it is important to talk it through with your doctor first.

Throughout the whole of the elimination diet you should keep a symptom diary, charting your symptoms, much as you have done when looking at pain and at your thoughts.

Exclusion phase

For two weeks you need to go on a diet consisting only of food from the following lists:

- Grains – rice and rice products, sago, tapioca, buckwheat products, millet products
- Proteins – veal, lamb, chicken, turkey, rabbit, tuna, trout or salmon, dried peas, lentils
- Fruit – peeled pears, peeled apples, pawpaw
- Vegetables – potatoes, sweet potatoes, lettuce, parsley, bamboo shoots, celery, cabbage
- salt – only a little!
- beverages – water, fresh pear juice

You may notice a flare up of symptoms in the first week, but generally it will settle down in the following week.

Challenge phase

Over the next two weeks you gradually include foods that you suspect cause you problems (e.g., wheat, milk and dairy products, alcohol and so on). If a food or drink does cause a problem it is likely to cause a flare-up in the next three or four hours, and the flare-up may go on for up to a couple of days. You do not take it again, but record it as a food to avoid.

If you notice no benefit to your symptoms by the end of four weeks it is unlikely that you will have any foods that are triggers and the diet can be stopped. If you have pinned down the foods that cause your problems, you may find that just eliminating them from your normal controlled diet will make a big difference.

The blood type diet

The blood type diet is an interesting diet that is based on the possibility that people with different blood groups fare better on some diets than others. The theory was established by Dr Peter D'Adamo, an American naturopathic physician, and his father, Dr James D'Adamo. I use this diet a great deal, and have found it very effective for some people, although it also can be quite restrictive, since it may require a person to have a different diet from everyone else in the home.

The thinking behind this theory is described below.

Blood group O

Blood group O represents man as a hunter. It is the oldest blood group. Type O people should:

- eat meat (high protein, low carbohydrate);
- avoid wheat and most grains; and
- exercise vigorously.

They will be prone to conditions like inflammatory arthritis if they eat the wrong foods. If they get arthritis they can get it in a more aggressive form.

Blood group A

Blood group A represents humans as they started to cultivate the land and grow crops. Type A people should:

- become vegetarian (high carbohydrate, low fat);
- engage in gentle pursuits, like walking, golf and yoga; and
- meditate and do relaxation exercises.

They are more prone to get osteoarthritis than rheumatoid arthritis.

Blood group B

Blood group B represents humans as nomads. Type B people can eat all the readily transportable foods that nomadic peoples can consume. They can eat the broadest diets – they may have meat and all dairy products, like cheese, but should avoid chicken. They should exercise moderately, such as by swimming, walking and gentle jogging. They may be prone to autoimmune disorders.

Blood group AB

Blood group AB represents modern humans, with all the strengths of their ancestors but their weaknesses as well. Type AB people should:

- use meditation and relaxing techniques; and
- take care to avoid living too fast.

They are likely to get osteoarthritis and degenerative ailments of modern life such as hypertension and heart disease.

If you wish to know more, Dr D'Adamo wrote his theories in *Eat Right 4 Your Type*, and also in *Arthritis: Fight it with the Blood Type Diet*. You will, of course, have to know your blood group. If you have had an operation, your doctor may be able to tell you. Women who have been pregnant will have been given their blood group on a card. Otherwise you may find out if you donate blood. Self-testing kits are also available.

The Mediterranean diet

To say that there is a Mediterranean diet is a bit misleading. Here I refer to a style of eating that is fairly typical of the region of the Mediterranean, but for which there is evidence that it is beneficial for health in general and also for arthritis and rheumatism.

This is a far easier diet to incorporate into daily life for more people than the blood type diet. It has the following characteristics:

- It contains high levels of fruits and vegetables, breads and other cereals, potatoes, beans, nuts and seeds.
- Olive oil is the only fat allowed.
- Moderate amounts of dairy products, fish and poultry are used, but very little red meat.
- Eggs are allowed, but no more than four a week and no more than one on any day.
- Wine is consumed in moderate amounts—two glasses per day for men, one glass for women.

The olive oil is very important, and I shall look at this in the section below on oils (see page 95); so too are the wine and the fruit and vegetables, all which are rich in anti-oxidants.

Improvement in symptoms, if they are to occur, may be seen within two to four weeks but can take up to three months. However, the Mediterranean diet is a healthy diet and it is worth considering for that alone.

Diets for gout

Gout has been known about for two millennia. In the past it was thought to be caused by excessive rich living, but it is now known to be the result of crystals of uric acid being deposited in the tissues and joints. If you reduce the purines and proteins in the diet this should make a difference. The main sources of purines are animal meat and seafood. Excess alcohol is also troublesome.

The diet should be structured around the following principles:

- Restrict red meat to reduce the purine levels, and replace it with low-fat or non-fat dairy products and soy products, such as soybeans and tofu.
- Make sure that dairy products are low in fat.
- Overall fat consumption should be limited to 30 per cent of the total calories consumed.
- Try to get your weight down towards a BMI of 25.
- Alcohol, especially beer, should be avoided.
- Drink plenty of fluids. Aim at drinking eight to ten 250 millilitre (eight fluid ounce) glasses of fluids, preferably water, each day.

One other thing I would suggest is to add cherries to the diet. If you have pain from gout, eat six to eight cherries a day. They can be in any form, fresh or frozen. This is a traditional Japanese treatment that seems to work.

Supplements

There are various things that you can take or add to your diet that may help. There is a confusing array of these, but I have restricted myself here to ones that I have used and found to be effective.

Oils

Everyone knows that you must not take too much fat into your system, and yet they hear about the benefits of various types of oils.

Understandably, there is a lot of confusion about fats and oils. I shall try to present this as simply as possible.

There are three basic types of fats – saturated, monounsaturated and polyunsaturated.

- Saturated fats are found in animal products such as meat, eggs, dairy products and seafood. In general these are considered 'bad' fats, since they have a tendency to push up your cholesterol and tend to promote inflammation. They do this because arachidonic acid, one of the fatty acids found in these fats, is broken down by enzymes into prostaglandins and leukotrienes, which are known to trigger inflammation.
- Monounsaturated fats are found in various nuts, including peanuts, walnuts and almonds, as well as in avocados and olive oil. They help to lower cholesterol and are 'good' fats, which can help to reduce inflammation.
- Polyunsaturated fats are the best fats, and are found in seafood and fish, corn oil and sunflower oil. They help to lower cholesterol and they are also anti-inflammatory. They are composed of two groups of essential fatty acids, called omega-3 and omega-6.

It gets more complicated than that. There are two types of omega-3s, those with long chains and those with short chains. The long chains are mainly found in oily fish. The two main ones are called eicosapentaenoic acid (EPA) and docosahexaenoic acid (DHA). These are anti-inflammatory and they have been found to be good for both arthritis and the heart. Short-chain omega-3s are found in foods like soya, flax, pumpkin seeds, walnuts and leafy green vegetables. They can be converted by the body into the long-chain fatty acids that do the most good.

You will find that lots of foods, like spreads, juices and even milk have added omega-3s. This is good in that the average British diet is really quite deficient in omega-3s. Yet the problem here is that it is more efficient to get the omega-3s in their natural form, that is from the oily fish, such as salmon, mackerel and sardines. Aim at having two or, even better, three portions of oily fish a week. But take care if you are prone to gout!

Olive oil, the only oil in the Mediterranean diet, contains no omega-3s. Its main constituent is oleic acid, which belongs to the omega-9 group. It is a bit of a mystery, but research is ongoing into its undoubted benefits. It certainly seems to have marked anti-inflammatory effects.

There is another group of fats, called trans fats, which are produced when oils have been hydrogenated. This process allows the oils to have a longer shelf life. You will find them in many packaged foods, French fries and microwavable popcorn. They are again 'bad' fats and are liable to promote inflammation.

So you see, the fats that you eat can either result in inflammation somewhere in your body, or reduce it. Essentially a diet rich in saturated fats, from meat and dairy products, will tend to promote inflammation and may well worsen arthritis, especially rheumatoid arthritis and the inflammatory arthropathies, and rheumatism. On the other hand, a diet rich in omega-3s from fish will reduce inflammation. Omega-6s also have anti-inflammatory benefits, but not as much as omega-3s, so you should try to get the balance in favour of Omega-3s.

Note that omega-3s inhibit blood clotting, so they 'thin' the blood. They should not be taken with aspirin or with anticoagulants. They should also be stopped two weeks before surgery. It is sensible to consult your doctor before taking them.

In general I prefer people to take the oils in foods, but you can try taking a supplement of fish oils containing ECA and DHA in a dose of 1,000 mg twice a day. They can bloat you, and some people find that they cause indigestion.

- Cod liver oil is derived just from the liver of the cod. It has omega-3s, but not as much as fish flesh. It does contain vitamin A and vitamin D. The latter helps you absorb calcium. It is a good anti-inflammatory agent in arthritis. The dosage is 500 mg to 1500 mg daily (one to three capsules), or a third of a teaspoon. However, care should be taken because the vitamin A can cause nausea and problems with vision. Cod liver oil should be avoided in pregnancy.
- Oil of evening primrose is rich in a fatty acid called gamma-linolenic acid (GLA). It has been shown to be effective in reducing inflammation in rheumatoid arthritis.
- Linseed oil or flaxseed oil are also worth trying and certainly seem to help some people. My own experience, however, is that they are not as effective as fish oil capsules.

Three anti-inflammatory spices

I think that it is worth considering using three spices in your cooking. They have all been shown to have anti-inflammatory properties and may help if used regularly. Take care, however, for they are heating herbs and can cause indigestion.

Curcumin

Curcumin is the active ingredient in turmeric that gives it the vivid yellow colour. It is also used to colour mustard powder. In trials it has been found as effective as hydrocortisone as an anti-inflammatory agent. Turmeric powder can be added to rice dishes, egg salad, salad dressings, curries, beans and sauces.

Ginger

The active ingredient of ginger is gingerol, a natural anti-inflammatory agent. It works by inhibiting some of the inflammatory prostaglandins, mentioned earlier. It can be taken as a supplement, in a dose of 500 mg to 1,000 mg daily. Alternatively, use powdered ginger on desserts or in baking.

Capsaicin

This is the active ingredient from cayenne or red chilli peppers. It is definitely known to have anti-inflammatory effects when taken in food. It is a hydrophobic substance, which means that it dislikes water and is not dissolved by water. This explains why drinking water will not relieve a burning mouth after eating chillies. All that water does is spread it around the mouth to make it worse, paradoxically. If you find yourself in such a situation, drink milk or a little alcohol, since capsaicin can be dissolved in fat (which milk contains) or alcohol.

It is also available over the counter or from your doctor as a rub-on agent for painful joints and muscles. It comes in two strengths and should be taken as your doctor suggests.

And three more useful supplements

Glucosamine sulphate and chondroitin sulphate

Glucosamine sulphate and chondroitin sulphate are both components of cartilage. In 2001 an important paper was published in the *Lancet* by a team from Belgium, Italy and the UK,[12] led by Jead Yves Reginster. They demonstrated in a three-year study that glucosamine sulphate markedly halted the progress of osteoarthritis and that it actually halted cartilage destruction. That is highly significant, because NSAIDs only reduce inflammation but do not have any effect in stopping progressive cartilage damage.

The effective dose of glucosamine sulphate is 1,000–2,000 mg daily. If it is taken on its own I usually suggest 500 mg three times a day. The effective dose of chondroitin sulphate is also 1,000–2,000 mg daily.

When the two are taken in combination, the lower dose of 1,000 mg for each seems to be adequate.

Glucosamine sulphate is derived from shrimp, crab and lobster shells. It must not, therefore, be taken by anyone who is allergic to seafood. It is also best avoided by anyone who is taking warfarin, since it may interact with the drug.

Chondroitin sulphate is derived from pork or beef cartilage. Both of them contain sulphate, so if you are allergic to sulphates you should avoid it.

WARNING If you have a seafood allergy, or you are taking warfarin, avoid anything derived from sea creatures.

Methylsulfonylmethane

Methylsulfonylmethane (MSM) is a good source of sulphur. This can be a wonder supplement to people who are low in sulphur – the problem being that there is no readily available test. I have found this to be very effective and people with very painful osteoarthritis and rheumatoid arthritis may be able to reduce their pain levels dramatically.

The dosage is 1,500–2,000 mg daily. Occasionally, people experience a worsening of symptoms for a week or two, but this is usually followed by improvement.

Minerals and vitamins

Vitamins B3, B5 and B6 reduce swelling of joints. Vitamin C is anti-inflammatory and vitamin E seems to improve flexibility. In addition, Vitamin D helps the body to absorb calcium.

I recommend my patients to take a good multi-vitamin and mineral supplement. Do check with your own doctor whether it is OK to take one if you are taking antihypertensive medication.

Key points

- Try to keep trim by adhering to some simple rules of thumb, such as getting your food intake right.
- Up to 50 per cent of people with arthritis and rheumatism may benefit from dietary manipulation.
- If your doctor agrees, take one of the anti-inflammatory oils.
- Consider adding the three anti-inflammatory spices to your diet.
- Consider taking a multi-vitamin and mineral supplement.

12

Complementary therapies

CAM (or complementary and alternative medicine) is the title given to a range of diverse practices that fall outside the remit of orthodox medicine. CAM includes homoeopathy, acupuncture, chiropractic, osteopathy, herbal medicine and reflexology. There is some blurring of margins nowadays since many GP practices offer one or more of these disciplines.

I have found the following therapies of benefit in my management of rheumatism and arthritis. This is not to say that other therapies that I have not mentioned will not help, but I have restricted myself to those that I have a good working knowledge of and that I believe people can incorporate into their self-help plan.

Progressive muscle relaxation

Progressive muscle relaxation is not really a complementary therapy at all, but a technique that is often used in hypnotherapy in order to deepen a state of relaxation. There is no great mystery about it and I recommend it to you if you have painful muscles from a condition like fibromyalgia. You may find it a big help.

Sit back in an easy chair or lie down somewhere that you will not be disturbed by a telephone or other interruptions. Take your shoes off. Close your eyes and just tell yourself that you are going to relax all your muscles. Tell yourself that as your muscles relax they will become less uncomfortable (use the word uncomfortable rather than painful).

Now clench your fists tightly for a count of seven. As you do this focus your attention on the tightness in the hands, feeling it increase as you count to seven. Suddenly let it go, and tell yourself that instead of tension there is now increasing relaxation in those muscles of the hand. And tell yourself that they will get even more relaxed as you count to 15.

Now clench your fists and tense the muscles of your feet by trying to clench the toes. Do this for a count of seven, exactly as before. Release suddenly and let the relaxation deepen for a count of 15.

Now clench all the muscles of your arms and of legs, in exactly the same way. Tense for seven and relax for 15.

Tense all the muscles of all your limbs, clench the buttocks together and tense the stomach muscles and your neck and face muscles. Screw your eyes tightly closed as you count to seven, and release suddenly and relax for 15.

Tell yourself that your muscles are now going to relax totally and that they will continue to relax and will feel more comfortable when you stop. Now imagine that a wave of relaxation is moving all the way up over your body from your feet, up your legs, up your back and chest to your neck. Let that feeling pass down both arms and up your neck to your head, relaxing all the muscles as it moves up over the top of your head and down over your face.

Tell yourself that you will enjoy that for a minute or so and that if you fall asleep, all well and good. But after the time is up just tell yourself that your muscles feel good and they continue to feel better, and that they will feel better each time that you do this.

It is as simple as that. And the thing is, the muscles will develop a memory and they will get less uncomfortable. Just make it something that you do every day.

Acupuncture and acupressure

Acupuncture has been practised in China for millennia. Traditionally, it is believed that energy flows along a series of 12 paired meridians or pathways and two special extra meridians. Imbalance of this energy flow can be rectified by the judicious insertion and stimulation of needles at indicated points. By contrast, Western medical acupuncture is based on physiological concepts including several of the ideas that I outlined in the chapter on pain. The nomenclature and numbering of the points used is common to both systems.

Western medical acupuncture works very well in many arthritic and rheumatic conditions. Up to 80 per cent of people will benefit to some degree. If you have no fears about having needle treatment, you may find that this is a worthwhile avenue of treatment.

You may still benefit from the phenomenon by trying some gentle acupressure on yourself. Use the pressure of the tips of the forefingers on the points and press in a gentle clockwise manner for half a minute to three minutes. Do the point on each side. Do this three times a day until you feel the condition ease. You will do no harm. This really is very simple; indeed much simpler than many books would have you believe. If the points are active they will be quite tender, and you may be

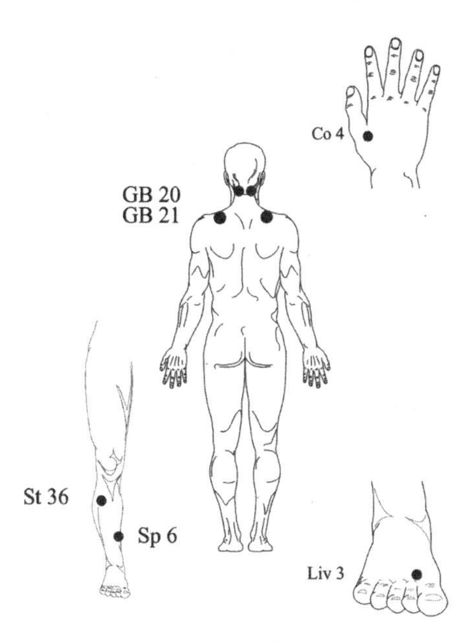

Figure 12.1 Some useful acupressure points

surprised at how effective they can be in easing pain. If so, you may find it worthwhile consulting a professional acupressure therapist or an acupuncturist. Many GPs now offer acupuncture as part of their practice.

The acupuncture points have an internationally agreed system of labelling. Each point is designated by two or three letters indicating a meridian (there are 12 meridians, each associated with an organ, plus two central meridians) and a number, starting at 1 and moving upwards. Thus, for example, Liv 3 means the third point on the liver meridian. I suggest using the six points as in Figure 12.1.

- Gall bladder 20 (GB 20) – you will find this easily, in a little hollow at the base of the skull about an inch from the midline on each side; for headache, neck pain, general upper body pains.
- Gall bladder 21 (GB 21) – another easy one to find, in the middle part of the trapezius muscle (if you put your hand on your opposite shoulder, the tip of the middle finger will probably be just over it); for shoulder pain, neck pain and back pain.
- Large intestine 4 or Colon 4 (LI 4 or Co 4) – in the web between the thumb and first finger; a point with many uses (toothache, jaw ache, hand pain, wrist pain, upper limb pain and abdominal spasms).
- Stomach 36 (St 36) – in the groove between the tibia and fibula; good for lower limb pains (e.g. arthritis of the hip or the knee), low

back and trunk pain, and surprisingly, sometimes very good for the shoulder.

- Spleen 6 (Sp 6) – four fingerbreadths up from the inside ankle bone (the medial malleolus), just behind the tibia; for lower limb problems, cramps, muscle pains, irritable bladder and period problems in women.
- Liver 3 (Liv 3) – in the web between the big and second toes; this has very similar properties to Co4 above. A good booster point for the immune system.

Osteopathy and chiropractic

These are two separate disciplines, although there is some overlap. They are both manipulation-based therapies dealing predominantly with the locomotor system. Chiropractors tend to focus on the joints of the spine, whereas osteopaths put just as much emphasis on the muscles, tendons and ligaments.

A good practitioner may be able to improve your mobility quite considerably over several sessions. They generally work in the private sector, although it is worth checking with your doctor as to whether they have contracted for these services. By law only someone registered with the General Chiropractic Council may use the title of chiropractor. Similarly, only those registered with the General Osteopathic Council can call themselves an osteopath.

Remedial massage

A registered practitioner in remedial massage treats only soft tissues. It is a gentler treatment than the manipulation offered by chiropractors and osteopaths, yet it may considerably help someone troubled with a rheumatic condition.

Reflexology

Reflexology is a therapy that involves treating, by a specific type of massage and manipulation, various reflex areas on the hands and feet. It does seem to get good results with various rheumatic symptoms. You may find that stimulating the reflex areas associated with the spine and the limbs can give you temporary relief. The areas corresponding to the spine are found along the inner arch of the feet, and areas corresponding to the limb girdles are on the outer side of the feet (Figure

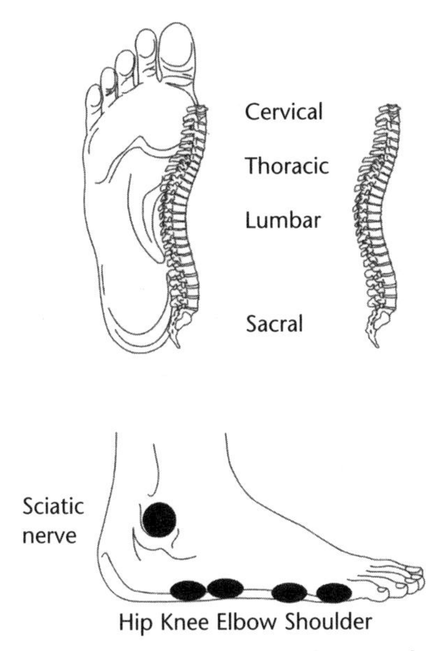

Figure 12.2 Reflexology: areas corresponding to the spine and limb girdles

12.2). A method that some people find helpful is to sit and roll a bottle or a cylinder back and forth on the floor with the appropriate part of the foot.

Homoeopathy

Homoeopathy is a gentle form of medicine based on the simile principle. The word 'homoeopathy' was coined by Dr Samuel Hahnemann (1755–1843) from the Greek words *homoios*, meaning 'similar' or 'like', and *pathos*, meaning 'suffering'. Essentially, this means that it is a therapeutic method using preparations of substances whose effects when administered to healthy subjects correspond to the manifestations of the disorder (the symptoms, clinical signs and pathological states). Most of the remedies, of which there are more than 4,000, are referred to by their Latin names.

Critics of homoeopathy have difficulty with the dilute states of the remedies used, believing that this dilution is the defining characteristic of the method. It is not – the defining characteristic is the simile principle, as explained above. The individual person's experience of the condition is of paramount importance, and the indicated treatment is the remedy that most closely matches the profile of the person's experience of their illness.

To get the most out of this method it is probably as well to see a qualified homoeopath. But, if you see that your pattern of symptoms matches one of these remedies, they are available to try yourself from most health shops, some chemists and all homoeopathic pharmacies.

Note that it is the pattern of the symptoms and the way that the person feels that is more important than the name of the condition.

- Rhus tox – for burning pain and stiffness that improves with movement, with heat (wheat bags, hot water bottle, etc) and with rubbing. Generally the symptoms are worse in cold and wet weather.
- Bryonia – for pains that are worsened by movement. Affected parts may get red, hot and swollen. Pressure seems to help, as does coldness, so that cold compresses and iced packs generally have been found to help.
- Kalmia – for shooting, tearing types of pain. They typically wander about and change. Thus they can move from the shoulders to the fingers and from the hips to the toes. Motion aggravates the pains.
- Ledum – for chilly people who paradoxically find that cold applications really help. Rheumatic pains tend to begin in the lower limbs and travel upwards. Very good for problems of the feet and ankles. Swellings of joints look pale, unlike the Bryonia picture.
- Rhododendron – for rheumatic pains that are worse in cold, damp weather and especially thunderstorms. The person may have an extreme fear of storms. Often causes pains about the shoulders.

There are different potencies available. In general, use a low potency such as a 6c and take one tablet twice a day until the symptoms settle. Alternatively, take a 30c potency twice a day for three days and wait to see if it improves. It can be repeated at two- or three-week intervals.

Herbal medicine

Herbal medicines can be very effective, but it is best to seek the opinion of a qualified herbalist. If you do, you should also tell your doctor that you are doing so, since it is important to know that you are not taking anything that could interact with your usual medication. This is extremely important in the case of Chinese herbs, since some of them have been shown to be toxic to the liver and kidneys.

You should also discuss with your doctor if you are considering taking anything like St John's wort (hypericum), since it can react with several orthodox medicines, including warfarin, cyclosporin, oral contraceptives, anticonvulsants, digoxin, theophylline and certain anti-HIV drugs.

The following herbs are certainly worth considering:

- Aloe vera, either taken as juice or as a capsule in a dose of 200 mg per day seems to be helpful in reducing pain, inflammation and stiffness.
- *Boswellia serrata*, or Indian frankincense, has been used in Ayurvedic medicine for many centuries. In the 1970s it was found to have anti-inflammatory properties that can help both osteoarthritis and rheumatoid arthritis as well as being helpful in inflammatory bowel disease. It can be effective as a cream to treat local inflammation, or by mouth to treat more extensive inflammation in a dose of 200 mg three times a day.
- Bromelain is a pineapple extract full of enzymes. It blocks the pathways of several of the body's chemical mediators of inflammation. I have had some success in reducing symptoms of rheumatoid arthritis with this. The dose is 250–500 mg twice a day.
- Nettle tea is a traditional remedy that does seem to help a good proportion of people. It is very bitter, however, and a little honey can take the edge off it. If you can manage two cups of it a day for a couple of weeks you may notice a difference.
- Quercetin is an extremely effective anti-oxidant that is found in apples, onions and tea. It may be the reason for the old adage 'an apple a day keeps the doctor away', since it does seem to be effective. I absolutely advise all my patients with arthritis and rheumatism to eat an apple every day.

Aromatherapy baths

The external use of oils has been used in medicine for millennia. It was an accidental explosion in the perfume laboratory of René Maurice Gattefossé in July 1910, however, that led to the development of aromatherapy. He severely burned his hands, but found that lavender oil had remarkable healing properties.

You should not massage essential oils directly onto the body. If you want to explore this therapy, and many people swear by it, visit a qualified aromatherapist.

You can, however, try a medicated bath, or a footbath if you are unable to get into a bath. For a bath, add six drops of the essential oil to a warm bath and relax in it for ten to 15 minutes. If using a footbath just use three or four drops and sit while you rest your feet in it for ten to 15 minutes.

The following essential oils are advocated as having pain-relieving qualities: bergamot, chamomile, lavender, marjoram and rosemary.

It is best to avoid aromatherapy if you are pregnant.

13

Myth or maybe?

Rheumatism and arthritis have attracted many folk remedies, sayings and myths. It is easy to be dismissive, yet often there is an element of truth that may lead to further fruitful research. It is worth looking at some of these topics, since you may want to make up your own mind about them.

'An apple a day keeps the doctor away'

The known health benefits of apples stretch back to antiquity. In the second century AD the famous Greek physician Claudius Galenus of Pergamum wrote that sweet apples aided digestion, and that sour apples were useful in people who fainted and in those who suffered from constipation. A thousand years later, a writer at the Medical School of Salerno, the first international medical school in the world, extolled the value of apples for rheumatism and for disorders of the bowels, the lungs and the nervous system.

I am not sure whether apples help in arthritis, yet I do think that there is good reason to have a daily apple. In 2001 the Mayo Clinic in the USA published a study that indicates that quercetin, a substance that is abundant in apples, helps to reduce the risk of prostate cancer. A later study by Cornell University in New York indicated that some chemicals in apple skins are capable of inhibiting the reproduction of colonic cancer cells by 43 per cent. Yet another, Finnish study indicated that diets with a high apple intake are associated with a 46 per cent reduction in the incidence of lung cancer.

Apples also seem to have a beneficial effect on the heart. In 1996 a Finnish study showed that people who ate apples regularly had a lower incidence of both heart disease and stroke. A California study recently indicated that two apples a day, or 350 millitres (12 fluid ounces) of apple juice, significantly reduce the damage caused by cholesterol.

So I do tend to advise an apple a day.

Copper bracelets

The use of copper bracelets to ease painful rheumatic conditions is said to go back to the ancient Greeks. Certainly, they are used by many millions around the world. You can buy them in jewellers', health shops and many sports shops. It has been postulated that tiny amounts of copper are absorbed through the skin and that this may in some way affect the body's inflammatory response to reduce the pain of various musculoskeletal conditions. Many professional sportsmen wear them.

A placebo-controlled trial involving 300 patients was reported in 1976.[13] The aim was to see whether people noticed any improvement in their symptoms, and to see whether there was a difference between wearing a copper bracelet or an aluminium bracelet that had been anodysed to look like copper. A significant number of people wearing the copper bracelets reported relief, as opposed to those who wore the dummy copper and those in the control group who wore no bracelet. In addition, the copper bracelets were found to have lost weight during the course of the trial, suggesting that some absorption of copper could have taken place.

This is the only trial that I was able to track down. It has not been replicated. However, the sheer number of people who wear them and feel that they help suggest that further research is indicated. This being the case, I think they are always worth a try.

Magnets

There are also a wide range of magnets available as jewellery, bands, insoles, studs and even mattresses. There is some evidence that suggests that they may help.

In 2004 a study was published in the *BMJ* (the *British Medical Journal*). Researchers from the Peninsula Medical School studied 194 patients aged between 45 and 80 years from five general practices in Devon, who had osteoarthritis of either the knee or the hip.[14] The patients were divided into three randomized groups and were asked to wear either a standard-strength magnetic bracelet, a weak magnetic bracelet or a 'dummy' or placebo bracelet. The trial lasted for 12 weeks, during which time the patients were asked to record scores on a recognized pain-scoring scale.

A significant difference was found between the standard magnetic bracelet group and the weak bracelet group. Indeed, the weak group recorded similar levels to the placebo group. The conclusion was that there was a recognized pain reduction in arthritis of the knee and hip when standard magnetic bracelets were worn, but that the strength of the magnet was important, needing to be 170 Tesla or greater. The researchers pointed out that they were uncertain whether the response was due to specific or non-specific effects.

This trial is not conclusive, but there is at least some evidence of efficacy. You can now also obtain copper magnetic bracelets. This does not mean that the copper is magnetized, since it is a non-magnetic element, but that magnets are contained in the copper bracelet. Again, this is worth a try.

The gin and raisin treatment

This one seemed to spread like an urban myth – that is, people seemed to hear about it from 'a man in a pub' or 'a friend of a friend'. Take a box of golden or white raisins (not dark ones) and soak them in gin in a flat container for a few weeks until the gin evaporates. Then take nine raisins a day, every day.

I have only heard anecdotes about this and have not met anyone who has tried it. Most accounts speak of the health benefits of grapes and the juniper from which gin is made, or the release of sulphur or sulphides. I am not convinced by this and have seen no evidence that it works. Certainly, people with gout should probably avoid it.

Should you avoid the nightshade family?

The *Solanum* or nightshade family includes tomatoes, potatoes, aubergines, and sweet and hot peppers. Dr Norman F. Childers, a horticulturist, advocated an avoidance diet and set up the Arthritis Nightshades Research Foundation. I am not convinced, and have not personally met anyone who seems to react to these foods. It is not an easy group to avoid and I do not suggest this to my patients. Yet it may work for you. Excluding them from your diet would do no harm. If you are going to do it, you would need to ensure that you exclude them totally, so a little reading up on the nightshades would be needed.

Does the weather affect people with rheumatism and arthritis?

This has almost become a joke in the same way that people with gout are always accused of high living. Many doctors say it is nonsense, yet patients report it time and time again, as I indicated in Chapter 12.

A study in 2004 from Barcelona looked at whether climate measures of humidity, pressure and temperature had any effect on arthritis.[15] They found that people with osteoarthritis experienced more pain when atmospheric pressure was low. People with rheumatoid arthritis experienced more joint pain when the temperature was low and less pain when it was high. So there seems to be a demonstrable change.

Epsom salts baths

Epsom salts baths are advocated by many to help the body to detoxify itself. Essentially, you apply the salts mixed with a little almond oil to the body from the neck down, avoiding the genital areas. You then soak in a tepid bath for five to ten minutes, wash off all surplus salts and towel yourself dry. It is important not to get up too quickly or you can feel dizzy. Have a drink of water and retire to bed. A perspiration reaction will occur and some staining of the pyjamas or nightclothes may be found in the morning.

This does seem to help some people, but it is not something to do very often – no more than twice a week. I am honestly not sure whether this does any more than a hot bath, with or without essential oils. It may be one to try and see for yourself.

Appendix: the Bach flower remedies

The main indications for the remedies in each group are listed below.

For fear

- Rock rose – for terror, panic, extreme fear.
- Mimulus – for fear of specific things, for example, illness, poverty, travelling, death.
- Cherry Plum – for fear of insanity or rash behaviour, including for impulsive, suicidal types who may live in fear of losing control.
- Aspen – for fears of unknown origin, such as dread, doom, fear that something dreadful is going to happen; people are often haunted by this fear, yet dare not confide in anyone.
- Red chestnut – for those who worry constantly that something will happen to their loved ones.

For uncertainty

- Cerato – for those who doubt their own judgement and who always have to ask others for their opinions.
- Scleranthus – quiet types who keep themselves to themselves, who find decisions difficult; their moods tend to fluctuate, as do many of their symptoms.
- Gentian – for those who are easily discouraged and who become dejected and despondent; any setback makes them feel disheartened.
- Gorse – for those who suffer utter despair and hopelessness and who don't believe that anything can be done to help.
- Hornbeam – for those who feel that they do not have enough strength, mentally or physically, to cope with what life throws at them, for whom everyday tasks seem too much, even though they can stir themselves to do them. These people feel that they need a helping hand. They may resort to stimulants. They commonly have a 'Monday morning' feeling.
- Wild oat – for the indecisive, who feel that they may have missed their way or have ended up in a rut and who cannot decide what to do for the future.

For unsufficient interest in present circumstances

- Clematis – for dreamy, inattentive people who seem to live in their own world, always dreaming about the future; they are unhappy with their own world and want to escape, and they may tend to feel faint.
- Honeysuckle – for those who live in the past.
- Wild rose – for those who just 'drift on' without making any effort to find joy or improve things and who become apathetic.
- Olive – for those who are drained of mental and physical energy, possibly because of past events or their condition; everything becomes an effort and they derive little pleasure from life.
- White chestnut – for those who cannot free themselves from some unwanted thought, which buzzes around in their mind; sleep may evade them because of it, and they can be mentally tortured by the thought.
- Mustard – for those who are subject to episodes of gloom and great sadness or depression; the feeling may fall like a curtain, dropping them into a black mood or depression for no obvious reason.
- Chestnut bud – for those who fail to learn from experience and who keep making the same mistakes.

For loneliness

- Water violet – for very quiet, independent people who like to be left to themselves in health or in illness; they can seem very aloof.
- Impatiens – for people with impatience and irritability and who want everything done in a hurry; they do not tolerate slowness in others; also good for general tension and stress, if you are 'taut like a band'.
- Heather – for the totally self-interested who seek any available company because they hate to be alone; they will unburden their problems on anyone.

For over-sensitiveness to influences and ideas

- Agrimony – for those who try to remain of cheery appearance, despite enduring inner torture; they may drink too much to cope.
- Centaury – for those who find it difficult to say 'no'; they let people ride rough-shod over them and may be timid and weak-willed.
- Walnut – for those who are bound to the past, family or habits by

strong links, and for those who need help coming to terms with life changes; this remedy is called the 'link-breaker'.

- Holly – for those who suffer from jealousy, suspicion, envy and anger; it is useful for strong negative emotions like 'hate'.

For despondency or despair

- Larch – for those who lack confidence and always expect to fail.
- Pine – for those who feel guilt and who blame themselves for everything.
- Elm – for those who feel overwhelmed by responsibility and who feel that they may have bitten off far more than they can chew.
- Sweet chestnut – for feelings of anguish, as if their limits of endurance have been passed and only oblivion and destruction is left.
- Star of Bethlehem – for the shock of bad news, fright after an accident, a bereavement and so on.
- Willow – for those who feel sorry for themselves.
- Oak – for those who struggle bravely on in the face of adversity, even though everything may seem hopeless; they get cross if illness interferes with their perceived duty of helping others.
- Crab apple – the cleansing remedy; for those who feel unclean and are disgusted; they are ashamed of their body and of their condition or illness.

For over-care for the welfare of others

- Chicory – for those who tend to be over-possessive; they want others to conform to their standards, and they may nag others and make martyrs of themselves; they may feign or exaggerate illness in order to maintain control over others.
- Vervain – for the fanatical, perfectionist and highly-strung who are rigid, tend never to change their views and want to convert others to their ways; they can get incensed by injustice.
- Vine – for the ruthless, domineering and tyrannical; they like power and they may make or have been good leaders.
- Beech – for critical and intolerant types; they tend to be arrogant.
- Rock water – for the self-disciplinarians who may be too hard on themselves; they may overwork and deny themselves things if their work is interrupted through 'flippancies'.
- The rescue remedy – for the emotional effects of shock; it consists of star of Bethlehem (for shock), rock rose (for terror and panic), impatiens (for tension and stress), cherry plum (for desperation) and clematis (for feeling faint).

Notes

1 Dr Samuel Smiles (1812–1904), Scottish doctor, social reformer and prolific author. His influential book *Self Help* was a Victorian best-seller.

2 Theophrastus Bombastus von Hohenheim (1493–1541), otherwise known as Paracelsus, was a medieval botanist, physician, surgeon and alchemist. He is credited with developing a mineral-based chemical approach to human health problems.

3 A pragmatic trial, on the other hand, looks at real-life situations and compares one treatment against another known treatment. These trials are used to determine whether the treatment works and is less concerned with the mechanism.

4 Pliny the Elder (23–79 AD), influential Roman writer and governor. He died of suffocation in 79 AD while making observations of the eruption of Mount Vesuvius, which destroyed Pompeii.

5 Claudius Galenus of Pergamum (131–201 AD), famed as Galen, was a Greek physician who worked in a gladiator school, later becoming physician to Marcus Aurelius. He was the first anatomist and the most influential medical writer for a thousand years.

6 The brain areas are made to 'light up' on a scan when the scan is used to measure and map the uptake of a chemical called FDG (fludeoxyglucose) in the brain. This is accepted as a good indicator of activity in the part of the brain that lights up.

7 Dr Hans Adolph Krebs was a German biochemist who described the Krebs cycle in 1937. He was awarded the Nobel Prize for Medicine in 1953. The Krebs cycle is also known as the tricarboxylic acid cycle (TAC) or the citric acid cycle, since citric acid is involved in the first step of the eight-part cycle.

8 Wolfe, F. The effect of smoking on clinical, laboratory, and radiographic status in rheumatoid arthritis. *Journal of Rheumatology* 2000; 27: 630–7; <www.jrheum.com/abstracts/abstracts00/630.html>.

9 Weingarten T.N., Podduturu V.R., Hooten W.M., et al. Impact of tobacco use in patients presenting to a multidisciplinary outpatient treatment program for fibromyalgia. *Clinical Journal of Pain* 2009; 25: 39–43.

10 Greendale G.A., Huang M.H., Karlamangla A.S., et al. Yoga decreases kyphosis in senior women and men with adult-onset hyperkyphosis: results of a randomized controlled trial. *Journal of the American Geriatrics Society* 2009; 57: 1569–79.

11 Body Mass Index is an accepted means of relating weight to height. It is easily worked out by dividing the weight in kilograms by the height in metres.

12 Reginster J.Y., Rovati L., Henrotin Y., et al. Long-term effects of

glucosamine sulphate on osteoarthritis progression: a randomised, placebo-controlled clinical trial. *Lancet* 2001; 357: 251–6.

13 Walker W.R., Keats D.M. An investigation of the therapeutic value of the 'copper bracelet'-dermal assimilation of copper in arthritic/rheumatoid conditions. Agents and Actions 1976; **6**: 454–9.

14 Harlow T., Greaves C., White A., et al. Randomised controlled trial of magnetic bracelets for relieving pain in osteoarthritis of the hip and knee. *BMJ* 2004; 329: 1450–4

15 Vergés J., Montell E., Tomàs E., et al. Weather conditions can influence rheumatic diseases. *Proceedings of the Western Pharmacology Society* 2004; 47: 134–6.

Useful addresses

Arthritis Care
18 Stephenson Way
London NW1 2HD
Tel.: 020 7380 6500;
0808 800 4050
(free confidential helpline)
Website: www.arthritiscare.org.uk

Arthritis Research Campaign
Copeman House
St Mary's Court
St Mary's Gate
Chesterfield
Derbyshire S41 7TD
Tel.: 0870 850 5000 (UK only);
+44 (0) 1246 558033
Website: www.arc.or.uk

Benefit Enquiry Line
Second Floor, Red Rose House
Lancaster Road
Preston
Lancs PR1 1HB
Tel.: 0800 882 200
Website: www.direct.gov.uk/en/D/1/Directories/DG_10011165

Disabled Living Foundation
380–384 Harrow Road
London W9 2HU
Tel.: 020 7289 6111
Helpline: 0845 130 9177 (10 a.m. to 4 p.m., Monday to Friday)
Website: www.dlf.org.uk

Fibromyalgia Association UK
PO Box 206
Stourbridge
West Midlands DY9 8YL
Tel.: 01384 895 002
Helpline: 0845 345 2322
Website: www.fibromyalgia-associationuk.org

National Wheelchair Managers' Forum
Website: www.wheelchairmanagers.nhs.uk/services.asp
This forum has set up the website to assist NHS managers involved in the provision of wheelchair services around the country. They have produced a Directory of NHS wheelchair services; these services provide appropriate mobility equipment for people of all ages with a long-term disability (i.e. likely to last longer than six months) who have difficulty walking. People running a particular local wheelchair service will help an individual to choose a wheelchair that best meets his or her needs. There is usually provision for short-term loan of wheelchairs (for those needing a wheelchair for less than six months).

Further reading

Craggs-Hinton, Christine, *Living with Fibromyalgia*. Sheldon Press, London, 2000.

D'Adamo, Peter J., *Eat Right 4 Your Diet*. New York, G. P. Putnam's Sons, 1996.

D'Adamo, Peter J., *Arthritis, Fight it with the Blood Type Diet*. London, Penguin, 2004.

Darlington, Gail, Gamlin, Linda, *Diet and Arthritis: a Comprehensive Guide to Controlling Arthritis through Diet*. London, BCA, 1998.

Hills, Margaret, *Curing Arthritis the Drug-free Way*. Sheldon Press, London, 1985.

Jarvis, D. C., *Folk Medicine*. Pan Books, London, 1971.

Jarvis, D. C., *Arthritis and Folk Medicine*. Pan Books, London, 1971.

Melzack, Ronald, Wall, Patrick D., *The Challenge of Pain*. 2nd edn. Penguin Books, London, 2008.

Souter, Keith, *Homoeopathy for the Third Age: Treatment for People in Middle and Later Life*. London, C. W. Daniels, 1993.

Souter, Keith, *Homoeopathy: Heart and Soul: Treatment for Emotional Problems*. London, C. W. Daniels, 1993.

Index